# The New Middle Ages

Series Editor
Bonnie Wheeler
English and Medieval Studies
Southern Methodist University
Dallas, TX, USA

The New Middle Ages is a series dedicated to pluridisciplinary studies of medieval cultures, with particular emphasis on recuperating women's history and on feminist and gender analyses. This peer-reviewed series includes both scholarly monographs and essay collections.

More information about this series at
http://www.palgrave.com/gp/series/14239

Tiffany A. Ziegler

# Medieval Healthcare and the Rise of Charitable Institutions

## The History of the Municipal Hospital

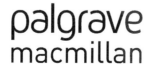

Tiffany A. Ziegler
Department of History
Midwestern State University
Wichita Falls, TX, USA

The New Middle Ages
ISBN 978-3-030-02055-2        ISBN 978-3-030-02056-9    (eBook)
https://doi.org/10.1007/978-3-030-02056-9

Library of Congress Control Number: 2018957443

© The Editor(s) (if applicable) and The Author(s), under exclusive license to Springer
Nature Switzerland AG, part of Springer Nature 2018
This work is subject to copyright. All rights are solely and exclusively licensed by the
Publisher, whether the whole or part of the material is concerned, specifically the rights
of translation, reprinting, reuse of illustrations, recitation, broadcasting, reproduction
on microfilms or in any other physical way, and transmission or information storage and
retrieval, electronic adaptation, computer software, or by similar or dissimilar methodology
now known or hereafter developed.
The use of general descriptive names, registered names, trademarks, service marks, etc. in this
publication does not imply, even in the absence of a specific statement, that such names are
exempt from the relevant protective laws and regulations and therefore free for general use.
The publisher, the authors and the editors are safe to assume that the advice and
information in this book are believed to be true and accurate at the date of publication.
Neither the publisher nor the authors or the editors give a warranty, express or implied,
with respect to the material contained herein or for any errors or omissions that may have
been made. The publisher remains neutral with regard to jurisdictional claims in published
maps and institutional affiliations.

Cover illustration: © Melisa Hasan

This Palgrave Pivot imprint is published by the registered company Springer Nature
Switzerland AG
The registered company address is: Gewerbestrasse 11, 6330 Cham, Switzerland

# CONTENTS

# CHAPTER 1

# Introduction

**Abstract** Before examining the history of the hospital and charitable institutions, it is first necessary to understand some key developments and terms. This introduction considers the important partnership between Christianity and institutional care, the rise of urbanization in the high Middle Ages and the problems it created, and the response—including the creation of hospitals—that popular Christian movements, such as the *vita apostolica activa*, brought. After a brief survey of the medieval hospital of Saint John in Brussels, I define the following terms: healthcare, disease, illness, hospitals, and *caritas*. The introduction concludes with a discussion of why historians must examine the hospital of Saint John in a greater history of charitable institutions.

**Keywords** Hospital of Saint John · Hospitals · Healthcare · Disease · Illness · *Caritas*

## INTRODUCTION

One of contemporary society's major concerns is healthcare; yet, healthcare is, and has always been, an age-old concept that has long plagued humankind. Queries often appear in today's news: should healthcare be public or private? If public, which public entities should care for the health of individuals: the state, religious groups, others? Should

© The Author(s) 2018
T. A. Ziegler, *Medieval Healthcare and the Rise
of Charitable Institutions*, The New Middle Ages,
https://doi.org/10.1007/978-3-030-02056-9_1

healthcare be free? What exactly constitutes healthcare? While some of these questions are difficult to answer—governments struggle on a daily basis to come up with solutions—others might be addressed by looking to history. Interestingly, the question of public versus private care is not new and not limited to modern medicine; it was one of many of the same problems that afflicted peoples of medieval society when it came to healthcare. While we may not be able to fully understand our current system of healthcare through a study of the Middle Ages, a systematic study of medieval healthcare and charitable institutions in the high Middle Ages, primarily from the perspective of the hospital, is a good place to start to look for answers.

This book is a systematic study of medieval healthcare and the rise of charitable institutions with a focus on the high medieval hospital. The purpose of this work is to introduce the institution of the hospital and society's obligation to care for those in need to a broad audience, as much of the work has previously been in the domain of specialists. Although the history of the hospital must begin with the rise of the first civilizations, which will be explored in the first chapters of this book, the history of the institution within its medieval context creates the basis for understanding the municipal hospital. The hospital of the Middle Ages, although analogous in many ways, took on a different character than their ancient predecessors and near eastern contemporaries: for Christian medieval societies, institutional charity was a necessity set forth by the religion's dictums—care for the needy and sick was a tenant of the faith, leading to a unique partnership between Christianity and institutional care. This partnership created a distinctive Christian hospital that would expand throughout the Middle Ages into the fledging hospitals of the early Modern period and the predecessors of today's institution.

## The Development of the Medieval Municipal Hospital

The medieval municipal hospital developed thanks to a unique combination of events that transpired in the Middle Ages. Beginning, in the early Middle Ages, monasteries and monks provided care for those who were sick and injured; their institutions served as pseudo hospitals.[1] Although

---

[1] The term pseudo hospital refers to those institutions that were designed for another purpose but still had or maintained a hospital. The monasteries of the early Middle Ages are prime examples of pseudo hospitals—they were monasteries first, while hospital care was one of many secondary obligations.

the main caregivers, monasteries were, by the twelfth century, overtaxed and burdened and could no longer support an increasing population in Europe.[2] By 1130, the Council of Clermont prohibited monks and clergy from practicing medicine. The high Middle Ages brought about a resurgence of trade and a blossoming of cities teaming with inhabitants: crowded in the confines of a city, the poor and sick became increasingly visible. For the first time since the fall of the Roman Empire, socially displaced poor and sick people began to plague the streets of European cities. These people were victims of the success of urbanization.[3] Recently forced both into despair and the view of the public through the loss of personal ties that had been a hallmark of village society, the displaced poor and sick became constant reminders that with all its wonders, urbanization also brought serious problems. Without monasteries, to whom would the poor and sick turn?

During the twelfth and thirteenth centuries, urbanization created a wonderful predicament in the towns and cities of Europe. Towns blossomed, and in many places, village settlements exploded into formidable cities.[4] While the immediate effects of urbanization included more croplands, better diets, increased trade and commerce, better learning, and an overall "renaissance,"[5] the long-term benefits were not always immediately realized. In the transition, a watershed occurred: traditional early medieval society had been classified as a "tripartite society" of those who pray, fight, and work.[6] The rise of cities, however, precipitated the

---

[2] Michel Mollat, *The Poor in the Middle Ages: An Essay in Social History*, trans. Arthur Goldhammer (New Haven: Yale University Press, 1986), 87.

[3] See especially, Lester K. Little, *Religious Poverty and the Profit Economy in Medieval Europe* (Ithaca: Cornell University Press, 1978).

[4] For more on the development of cities throughout Europe, see David Nicolas, *The Growth of the Medieval City: From Late Antiquity to the Early Fourteenth Century* (New York: Routledge, 1997, 2014), and for the region of Brussels, see Alexandre Henne et Alphonse Wauters, *Histoire de la Ville de Bruxelles* (Bruxelles, 1968); and Ernest Smith, *The Story of Brussels* (Didactic Press, Kindle Edition, 2014).

[5] See Charles Homer Haskins, *The Renaissance of the Twelfth Century* (Cambridge: Harvard University Press, 1927).

[6] Traditionally, this phrase is attributed to one of two sources. The first comes from Bishop Aldabero of Laon on 1027/31. The second author is Bishop Gerard I (1012–51), a canon of Cambrai on 1023/4 and the bishopric from which the hospital of Saint John would later receive its statutes. Within one hundred years, the social structure would fall into transformation, making the distinction of three classes void. For more on both men, see Giles Constable, *Three Studies in Medieval Religious and Social Thought* (Cambridge: Cambridge University Press, 1998), 283–284.

growth of trade and commerce, and created professions for which the traditional divisions did not account, i.e., merchants and burghers.[7] This new merchant-burgher class not only challenged the bounds of tripartite society and created a social upheaval, but also began to dictate a new set of social norms.[8]

As society moved from a land-based economy and barter society to a cash society, lands and rents once limited to only the upper nobility became available to lesser nobles, who were now able to participate in some of the more earmarked customs and traditions, especially in regard to land donations. Armed with lands and rents and motivated by the visible crowds of the sick and poor, an explosion in lay piety via land donations thus coincided with urban developments and provided much-needed help in the immediate period. Men and women alike sought out a life inspired by that of Christ Jesus and his Apostles (*vita apostolica activa*).[9] They took to heart Jesus' Sermon on the Mount, "Blessed of are the poor...,"[10] while those who had provided care would find eternal salvation, thanks to the biblical dictum, "I was sick and you took care of me."[11]

Renewed care for the poor and sick continued to be an expression of Christ's compassion for those too weak to care for themselves and was initially introduced to municipal areas with poor tables, confraternities, *leprosaria*, and monastic hospitals, which were created to feed, clothe, provide shelter for, and heal those in need. Although religious institutions were largely tied to the dissemination of goods and care, changes in

---

[7] See Georges Duby, *The Early Growth of the European Economy: Warriors and Peasants from the Seventh to the Twelfth Century* (Ithaca: Cornell University Press, 1978).

[8] See Henri Pirenne, *Medieval Cities: Their Origins and the Revival of Trade*, trans. Frank D. Halsey (Princeton: Princeton University Press, 1925, 1969, 1975).

[9] See, for more on the concept of *vita apostolica activa*, Little, *Religious Poverty and the Profit Economy in Medieval Europe* and Mollat, *The Poor in the Middle Ages: An Essay in Social History*. Although mendicants and laymen alike were encouraged to live a life like that of Christ Jesus or his apostles, they could also follow the apostolic example of women like Mary and Martha. For more on this notion, see Katherine Ludwig Jansen, *The Making of the Magdalen: Preaching and Popular Devotion in the Later Middle Ages* (Princeton: Princeton University Press, 2000). Many of the concepts outlined in these works have been nicely condensed by Adam J. Davis, "The Social and Religious Meanings of Charity in Medieval Europe," *History Compass*, Vol. 12, No. 12 (December 2014): 935–950.

[10] Matthew 5:3 RSV.

[11] Matthew 25:36 RSV.

society and the economy provided for greater lay participation, especially after monasteries were forbidden to provide medical care.

Subsequently, the urban center became a breeding ground for charitable and medicinal care,[12] especially in the thirteenth century with the rise in Mariological devotion. The thirteenth century witnessed increasing reliance on the Virgin Mary as the Mother of Mercy (*mater misericordiae*) and as an intercessor between Christ and sinners. This trend solidified the concept of love of neighbor as opposed to love of God. The suffering Christ was replaced with Christ on judgment day who would judge men and women. The average Christian could only hope to please this new Christ through the human and understanding Virgin Mary and through charitable care of one's neighbors. Institutions—poor tables, confraternities, *leprosaria*, etc.—thus appeared throughout the bourgeoning cities. It was, however, the medieval hospital that became the ideal repository for the gifts of the concerned classes.

While civic and municipal hospitals arose all throughout Europe, one of the defining locations for the hospital movement was in the modern city of Brussels where a particular institution, the hospital of Saint John, arose to become an excellent example of the medieval municipal hospital. Brussels, specifically, and the Low Countries in general, were some of the first places to address the new urban issues systematically. By the twelfth century, Brussels had several hospitals, a leprosarium, poor tables, and even the remnants of monastic hospitals. While the existence of many institutions could seem like what has been called the "private" and

---

[12]The crisis of urbanization not only precipitated social and communal evolutions but also new social and institutional structures, many of which came as responses by local churchmen and nobles, in addition to burghers and merchants, to remedy the unforeseen urban problems. Several scholars have identified these trends in areas throughout Europe, including Edward J. Kealey in his social history of Anglo-Norman medicine in the twelfth century and Sharon Farmer in her study on the poor men and women of thirteenth- and fourteenth-century France. Edward J. Kealey, *Medieval Medicus: A Social History of Anglo-Norman Medicine* (Baltimore: The John Hopkins University Press, 1981). Sharon Farmer, *Surviving Poverty in Medieval Paris: Gender, Ideology, and the Daily Lives of the Poor* (Ithaca: Cornell University Press, 2002, 2005). While both these and other works demonstrate that significant advances are being made in the study of the poor and the institutions created for them after the crisis of urbanization, there are still many gaps in scholarship, including coverage of the Low Countries in general and twelfth- and thirteenth-century Brussels specifically.

"*ad hoc* nature of medieval charity,"[13] it was, rather, the basis for centralized care. The hospital of Saint John in Brussels began as the typical private hospital, but later, it evolved into a municipal hospital to provide centralized care.

A brief survey of the pivotal changes shows this very evolution. In 1186, Roger, the Bishop of Cambrai, first approved the foundation of a charitable confraternity in honor of the Holy Spirit. The confraternity, made up of a triad of priests, clerics, and "*bourgeois*,"[14] and located in Brussels, was the future hospital of Saint John.[15] In 1195, the hospital of the Holy Spirit began to take shape: its main mission was care for retirees.[16] Sometime between 1195 and 1204, the hospital's name changed from the Holy Spirit to Saint John, while care slowly shifted away from retirees to the general public.[17] While it is not fully clear from the extant records, early hospital care and management was provided by a small number of brothers: Pope Innocent III on August 3, 1207 placed the brothers of the hospital and their holdings under the protection of the papacy.[18] Four years later, the hospital added sisters to their ranks, as they were needed to tend to the infirm too sick to beg, women lying in,

---

[13] Sharon Farmer, "From Personal Charity to Centralised Poor Relief: The Evolution of Responses to the Poor in Paris, c. 1250–1600," in *Experiences of Charity*, ed. Anne M. Scott (Burlington: Ashgate, 2015), 42.

[14] This is the title given in the introduction to the charter. The word used is *burgensibus*. What is meant by the translation is not *bourgeoisie*, but rather the townsmen, particularly those of aldermen status. This makes sense in the hospital's later history, as the town aldermen played a particularly important role in the institution and its affairs. For more on Brussels' aldermen, see Alphonse Wauters, "Les Plus Anciens Écevins de la ville de Bruxelles," *Annales de la Société d'Archéologie de Bruxelles: Mémoires, Rapports et Documents*, tome 8 (Bruxelles, 1894).

[15] *Cartulaire de l'Hôpital Saint-Jean de Bruxelles (Actes des XIIᵉ et XIIIᵉ Siècles)*, ed. Paul Bonenfant (Brussels: Palais des Académies, 1953), SJ 2, pp. 5–7. The original is lost.

[16] *Cartulaire de l'Hôpital Saint-Jean*, SJ 4, pp. 8–10. The original is lost. Duke Henry I (1165–1235), in order to encourage bequests and donors, drew up an exemption in 1195 from military obligations for those who would retire to the hospital. Retirees would be liable for their payments on their fiefs and could no longer engage in their secular trades or pursuits, while the hospital would inherit their estates.

[17] *Cartulaire de l'Hôpital Saint-Jean*, SJ 5, pp. 10–13. CPAS, SJ 4.

[18] "*fratribus hospitalis Brucellensis*." *Cartulaire de l'Hôpital Saint-Jean*, SJ 6, pp. 13–14. CPAS, SJ 4.

and orphaned children, all under the institution's care.[19] By October of 1211, John III, Bishop of Cambrai, granted Saint John's hospital its statutes of 37 articles.[20]

In approximately twenty-five years, the hospital went from a private confraternity and retiree community to a centralized general hospital,[21] which was a fairly typical occurrence. Its statutes specified the care that was to be given to pregnant women and orphaned children, to those too ill to beg, and to those too sick to care for themselves, falling in line with the reform councils of the early thirteenth century. In the transition, it became clear that this was no longer a private hospital: it was a centralized public one. It is thus without surprise that the hospital increased in size and renown throughout the 1200s. The hospital's foundation, special mission of care, and development—linked to a triad of responsible parties and a key location—created a remarkable and unusual atmosphere for Saint John hospital to grow.

Moreover, Saint John hospital stood at the center of the town, nearly equidistant from all the major urban centers: the market, the ducal palace, and the cathedral chapter. This location placed the hospital at the center of the town and town life. The duke of Brabant, the bishop of Cambrai, the dean of the cathedral of Saint Gudule, the town aldermen, the town castellan, the merchants and businessmen, and even the preverbal butcher, baker, and candlestick maker saw the hospital when they went about their days. Yet, these very peoples also saw the poor and sick recently brought into view by the effects of urbanization. Viewing those less fortunate, while being casually reminded of the place that could help the sick, prompted Brussels' inhabitants to provide graciously to the hospital of Saint John in a fashion that can only be described as centralized.

---

[19] The sisters too are noted in the charters: a 1209 document addresses the "*fraters et sorores hospitalis beati Johannis in Bruxella.*" See *Cartulaire de l'Hôpital Saint-Jean*, SJ 7, pp. 15–16. The original is lost.

[20] *Cartulaire de l'Hôpital Saint-Jean*, SJ 10, pp. 19–25. The original is lost.

[21] A general hospital can be used to describe a large institution that often results for the consolidation of smaller institutions. Saint John hospital seems to fit this definition when one considers that it started as a confraternity, served the retirees of the community, and then eventually transitioned to care of all individuals in need. While not as large as some of its contemporaries, it was large enough to serve the needs of Brussels. Furthermore, a general hospital is one that is open to the public. Saint John hospital and Saint Pierre Leprosarium were the only institutions to serve this need in Brussels. For more on the size of the hospital, its inmate population, and more see Chapter 5 of this work.

While its location ensured that all peoples from across the social spectrum frequented the institution, it was the changes in the period and the hospital's creation that further set it apart from its counterparts. The economic and religious advancements of the period led to the creation and support of a largely *urban* institution. Tied to the rise of cities, the development of pseudo-healthcare, the changes to the profit economy, and the arrival of mass congregations of poor and sick to the urban centers of Europe, the hospital became the new "urban monastery" and the new recipient of charitable donations. Not only did it serve as Brussels' municipal hospital, it also went on to serve as a model for neighboring institutions. The hospital of Saint John took on a new character that the other Brussels' institutions lacked: its care was overreaching, and it could provide for a number of maladies and conditions.[22] Yet, the concern for *caritas* never left the institution. From its creation as a confraternity, to its reception of a chapel, to its donations from peoples from all stations in Brussels, the hospital of Saint John was the epitome of charitable healthcare, which, despite clear evolutions in medical practices, I would like to believe, we still see today.

## DEFINITIONS

What I am thus proposing is that we can learn about healthcare and its application in today's world by studying medieval hospitals in general and Saint John hospital in Brussels specifically. In particular, we can see the rise of the general hospital with a mission of care for all in the high Middle Ages that extends to the present day. Direct comparisons, however, are difficult, and in an attempt to not be anachronistic, I will be working from some basic definitions for the terms healthcare, disease, illness, hospitals, and *caritas*.

In a modern sense, healthcare is a blanket term for the care of individuals via diagnosis and treatment.[23] Healthcare seeks to improve physical and mental conditions, illnesses, diseases, and injuries, while healthcare professionals, such as physicians, nurses, dentists, midwifes, pharmacists, and more all play key roles in the delivery of various treatments.

---

[22] Care at the hospital included everything from administering basic treatments, to providing for children and orphans, to helping women in their laying in periods and during birth, to providing hospice care.

[23] Sometimes prevention is also included as an element of healthcare.

Treatments range for medicinal (i.e., medical care or professional treatment as dictated by the guidelines of the professional medical community), to herbal, to therapeutic, and beyond. Healthcare in the modern world tends to be an all-encompassing approach to the well-being of an individual.

Modern healthcare can be neatly divided into two categories: public or private. Public healthcare is a "field that seeks to improve lives and the health of communities through the prevention and treatment of disease and the promotion of healthy behaviors such as healthy eating and exercise."[24] Typically, the government of a particular community provides public healthcare, while private healthcare falls to private entities. Both private and public institutions of healthcare work in a holistic way to ensure the health of an individual against disease and illness.

If, however, healthcare is designed to protect against disease and illness and to treat the complications that arise from disease and illness, we must consider what exactly disease and illness are. Kenneth M. Boyd explains, "concepts such as disease and health can be difficult to define precisely. Part of the reason for this is that they embody value judgments and are rooted in metaphor. The precise meaning of terms like health, healing and wholeness is likely to remain elusive, because the disconcerting openness of the outlook gained from experience alone resists the reduction of first-person judgments (including those of religion) to third-person explanations (including those of science)."[25] The definitions Boyd gives come from the modern medical practitioner, and then they are distilled further to consider issues of value judgments, metaphors, and religion. As a result, the tidy explanations follow: "disease then, is the pathological process, deviation from a biological norm. Illness is the patient's experience of ill health, sometimes when no disease can be found. Sickness is the role negotiated with society."[26]

Within each of these definitions exists a sense of locality and bodily presence. Disease and illness are experienced in the body, while sickness is the state of the body as a person interacts with society. This is

---

[24] Healthcare.gov, "Public Health Care," accessed 19 September 2017 at https://www.healthcare.gov/glossary/public-health/.

[25] Kenneth M. Boyd, "Disease, Illness, Sickness, Health, Healing and Wholeness: Exploring Some Elusive Concepts," *Journal of Medical Ethics: Medical Humanities*, Vol. 26 (2000): 9–17, here 9.

[26] Boyd, 10.

a modern concept; the body was not always believed to be an origin of disease. Such notions developed later in modern history, and in his study on the birth of modern medicine, Michel Foucault notes that "the space of *configuration* of the disease and the space of *localization* of the illness in the body have been superimposed, in medical experience, for only a relatively short period of time—the period that coincides with nineteenth-century medicine and the privileges accorded to pathological anatomy."[27] If we are to believe in the localization of disease and illness, we need to thus consider the places for which people can receive care for the body, namely the clinic, and before modern practices, the hospital.

The hospital as a so-called "therapeutic instrument, as an instrument of intervention of illness for the patient, an instrument capable either along or through its effects, of curing" is a "relatively modern concept, dating from the end of the eighteenth century."[28] This idea regarding the exclusive modernity of hospitals is primarily because of works like those of Foucault who argued that the hospital was a "means of intervention on the patient,"[29] and that the "architecture of the hospital must be the agent and instrument of cure."[30] Prior to the modern hospital, Foucault argued that early modern and medieval hospitals were where patients were sent to die.[31] Although there is some truth in this—the medieval hospital was at times a hospice where the sick or aged could live out the remainder of their lives in comfort—it is not the whole truth. Indeed, the medieval hospital provided a "mixture of functions of assistance and spiritual transformation which were incumbent upon the hospital. These were the characteristics of the hospital until the beginning of the eighteenth century."[32] Thus, we must ask, was the medieval hospital really that different?

---

[27] Michel Foucault, *The Birth of the Clinic: An Archeology of Medical Perception*, trans. A. M. Sheridan Smith (New York: Vintage Books, 1973, 1994), 3–4.

[28] Léopold Lambert, *The Funambulist*, "Foucault Episode 6: Architecture and Discipline: The Hospital," accessed 22 September 2017 at https://thefunambulistdotnet.wordpress. com/2012/06/29/foucault-episode-6-architecture-and-discipline-the-hospital/.

[29] Michel Foucault, "La politique de la santé au XVIIIe siècle," in *Les Machines à guérir, Aux origines de l'hôpital moderne*, dossiers et documents (Paris: Institut de l'environnement, 1976), 11–21.

[30] Michel Foucault, "La politique de la santé au XVIIIe siècle."

[31] Ibid.

[32] *Space, Knowledge and Power: Foucault and Geography*, eds. Jeremy W. Crampton and Stuart Elden (New York: Ashgate/Routledge, 2016), 144.

Perhaps the medieval hospital was not only similar to but the basis of our modern system today. As we transition to examine how these same terms were defined in the Middle Ages, we run into some problems. The issue in trying to define healthcare for the Middle Ages, or really for any time before the modern period, is that the definition varies and is not always as precise. This is largely because knowledge in the medical field was not necessarily consistent or comprehensive. There was a clear difference, for example, between medicine and literate medicine. Monica H. Green, in her examination of the *Trotula* texts, a compendium on women's medicine, explains,

> The history of the *Trotula* was played out on a terrain somewhere between the high learned medicine of the universities and the wholly oral practices of illiterate empirics. I call this terrain 'literate medicine', the realm of medical thought and practice that involves medical knowledge that has been written down, knowledge that has been committed to a textual and not simply oral mode for its transmission. 'Literate medicine' is a much broader category than learned medicine (for example, the formal commentaries and scholastic disputations of the universities), which will demand competence not only with a large technical vocabulary but also with sophisticated philosophical concepts for its interpretation. Literate medicine encompasses learned medicine, of course, but it also includes written material such as recipes jotted down in the back of a notebook or a little handbook of daily regimen.[33]

Taken a step further, some would argue that healthcare treatment via modern medical procedures cannot be compared to the practices of the pre-modern period. Monica H. Green, queries, for example, "whether our field generally should continue to define itself as a history of medicine, or rather as a history of *health (sic)*," noting the benefits of equating the two.[34]

---

[33] Monica H. Green, *Making Women's Medicine Masculine: The Rise of Male Authority in Pre-modern Gynaecology* (Oxford: Oxford University Press, 2008), 12. See also Monica H. Green, "Gendering the History of Women's Healthcare," *Gender & History*, Vol. 20, No. 3 (2008): 487–518.

[34] Monica H. Green, "'History of Medicine' or 'History of Health'," *Past and Future*, No. 9 (Spring/Summer 2011): 7.

Even with such degree of differences, the fact of the matter was that care was present in the Middle Ages and even sought out. Again, Monica H. Green explains that there was

> slight evidence that there was a growing general belief in the ability of learned medicine to provide desirable medical care. In monasteries and nunneries, which ever since the time of Benedict had been expected to run their own infirmaries to care for their sick, there is widespread evidence for the employment of professional practitioners from outside the community to tend to their more grievously ill. These communities sometimes even signed contracts with licensed practitioners to ensure their attendance when needed. Lay people as well, from the nobility to the middling urban classes, sought out the ministrations of learned practitioners and signed contracts with them to ensure their availability.[35]

Obviously, professional healthcare existed in the Middle Ages, and while some might classify what the monks and the lay hospital staff performed as 'hospitality', it is clear that professionalism at an institution of sorts was employed.

Moreover, the terms hospitality and healthcare were not necessarily mutually exclusive in the Middle Ages. Hospitality focuses on the reception of guests, be it friends, acquaintances, or strangers who are received kindly and graciously, whereas the word hospital is derived from *hospes*, a host or guest.[36] During the Middle Ages, hospitals were created, similar to what Foucault would argue, to respond to social needs; the motives were *always* religious in origin, thus signifying the importance of the root of the word of hospitality in a Christian context.[37] In this sense, hospitality and healthcare cannot be separated from each other; doing so becomes an "arbitrary practice of historians to divide the study of religious experience from the rest of daily life."[38]

This is why the study of medieval hospitals is murky at times. Many medieval hospitals were created to care for the infirm and aged people; they were indeed places that people went to die. Yet, as noted by Rotha

[35] Monica H. Green, *Making Women's Medicine Masculine*, 7–8.

[36] Rotha Mary Clay, *The Medieval Hospitals of England* (London: Frank Cass, 1966), 1.

[37] Pierre de Spiegeler, *Les Hôpitaux et l'Assistance à Liège (Xe-Xve Siècles): Aspects Institutionnels et Sociaux* (Paris: Sociéte d'Edition "Les Belles Lettres," 1987), 47.

[38] Lisa M. Bitel, *Women in Early Medieval Europe 400–1100* (Cambridge: Cambridge University Press, 2002), 95.

Mary Clay, "such a home was called indiscriminately 'hospital,' 'Maison Dieu,' 'almshouse' or 'bedehouse,'"[39] suggesting that both care in a medical sense and hospitality were provided. In addition, control of a hospital varied. Sometimes, there was municipal control of a hospital, and sometimes control was connected to a local trustee, while almost all were under the auspice of the local bishop.[40] Here in particular, it is hard to separate public and private care. Western cities, their governments, and their trustees were primarily Christian. There were also guild almshouses and private almshouses, while there were separate hospitals for Jews, homes for poor clergy, and for lay "gentlefolk."[41] In addition, hospitals for women and children, lepers, and the insane also existed. While a private entity might over see the hospital and its care, it was always tied to religion. As a result, the "hospital was a semi-independent institution, subject to royal and Episcopal control in matters of constitution, jurisdiction and finance, yet less trammeled in organization than most religious houses. It formed a part of the parochial system, and had also links of one kind or another with monastic life;"[42] to remove the aspects of hospitality, religion, or charity from the medieval hospital would make for an incomplete argument.

## COMPARISONS

If so different in many ways from their modern counterparts, how do we compare the medieval institutions to the modern hospital? For this, we look to what seems to be the foundation of every hospital regardless of origin, organization, governance, and more. The defining characteristic of the medieval hospital was *caritas*. The Latin root of *caritas* traces the definition back to something of "dearness, costliness, high price" in association with objects that were highly valued.[43] The meaning eventually evolved to include "regard, esteem, affection, [and] love" in a more brotherly sense,[44] while *caritates* were "the loved persons."[45]

---

[39] Rotha Mary Clay, *The Medieval Hospitals of England*, 15.

[40] Rotha Mary Clay, *The Medieval Hospitals of England*, 17.

[41] Rotha Mary Clay, *The Medieval Hospitals of England*, 23.

[42] Rotha Mary Clay, *The Medieval Hospitals of England*, 211.

[43] *A Latin Dictionary*, "*caritas*," eds. Charlton Lewis and Charles Short (The Clarendon Press and Oxford University Press, 1962), 292. See use, for example, by Cicero and Cato.

[44] Lewis and Short, *A Latin Dictionary*, 292.

[45] Ibid.

The definition continued to change as time went on, and the addition of Christianity in the Roman Empire transformed the meaning once again: "In a broad sense, charity comes to denote an affection that is nonphysical and directed primarily toward God. From this love of God flows a warmth toward other human beings: friends, strangers, and even enemies."[46] This 'warmth' and the display of such warmth closely mimic the definition of hospitality. Furthermore, "this caring for others can have many expressions: group solidarity and a spirit of brotherhood, personal friendship, or a sense of individual contentment."[47] Never was this more present than at the medieval hospital, especially with the increased focus on the Virgin Mary in the thirteenth century. She became the advocate for compassion and care for those who could not provide for themselves.

The medieval hospital provided healthcare via hospitality, and by extension, it delivered *caritas*. Although much has changed, a sense of care is still embodied at the modern institution. Differences remain, yet there are still some holdovers. Secular care provided by the medieval institution cannot be separated from the spiritual care that occurred. Indeed, all hospitals were founded with a chapel.[48] Many modern hospitals have a chapel in them. In addition, the medieval hospital served both the body and soul. Sin and disease were not necessarily distinct and could often be equated with each other. Disease could even be a sign of a greater sin, and thus care for the soul and body. The approach taken was thus holistic. This was a departure from the monastic hospital that was mainly designed as a hospice. The intent was to heal in *every* way

---

[46] James William Brodman, *Charity and Religion in Medieval Europe* (Washington, DC: The Catholic University of America Press, 2009), 3.

[47] James Brodman, *Charity and Religion in Medieval Europe*, 2–3. According to James Brodman, "charity exhibits several characteristics. First of all, it implies an altruism toward humanity, or at least toward those within society who were regarded as vulnerable, degraded, or in serious material need. [...] Secondly, the concern for others is motived by a spirit that has a religious character and no merely one designed to preserve a particular social order by, for example, pacifying the poor. [...] Finally and significantly, medieval religious charity was highly fragmented an inchoate; it never coalesced into a coherent or cohesive organization."

[48] The chapel was a major source of income to the hospital; many donors made contributions on the condition that masses would be celebrated for them. See Pierre de Spiegeler, *Les Hôpitaux et l'Assistance à Liège*, 193–194.

possible. These factors made the medieval hospital unique; it was an embodiment of several notions that combined to make one institution from which we get the modern hospital. I think it would be a mistake to say that hospitals today do not take a holistic approach.[49]

*Medieval Healthcare and the Rise of Charitable Institutions: The History of the Municipal Hospital* is the history of the development of medieval institutions of care, beginning with a survey of the earliest known hospitals in ancient times to the classical period, to the early Middle Ages, and finally to the explosion of hospitals in the twelfth and thirteenth centuries.[50] In this study, the hospital of Saint John in Brussels serves as the example of the developments. Saint John's hospital in Brussels was not only vital to the people of the city; it became a model for later medieval municipal hospitals. The institution followed the pattern of the establishment of medieval charitable institutions in the high Middle Ages, but later diverged to become the archetype for later Christian hospitals.

[49] Many hospitals offer alternative therapies, from acupuncture, to energy healing, to yoga studios.

[50] To say that a history of charitable institutions and/or hospitals in the Middle Ages does not exist would be a lie. There are several histories, but those histories do not reveal the whole picture, especially in regard to hospitals. James Brodman's *Charity and Religion in Medieval Europe* has made a phenomenal contribution to the field, especially in the context of lay generosity, charitable institutions, and religious support by the papacy. Brodman places new emphasis on the active role of the laity, detailing lay involvement in various charitable institution—including the hospital of Saint John in one chapter. Paramount, however, to understanding the further development of charitable institutions into hospitals is the urban milieu. The changes undergone by the laity, as Brodman highlights, are religious in nature, so much so that he sees religion as the only basis for a coherent movement in medieval society. He describes society's response to charity as "highly fragmented and inchoate" arguing that it "never coalesced into a coherent or cohesive organization;" charity tended to be localized. Brodman, *Charity and Religion in Medieval Europe*, 2–3. While I find the assessment of religious charity correct, the idea of a fragmented, incoherent concern for the poor ignores societal, economic, and urban structural evolution. Many scholars, such as Sharon Farmer described above, are turning to this idea, as it is within the multiple transitions that the centralized municipal hospital was born. Sharon Farmer, "From Personal Charity to Centralised Poor Relief: The Evolution of Responses to the Poor in Paris, *c.* 1250–1600," in *Experiences of Charity*, ed. Anne M. Scott (Burlington: Ashgate, 2015), 42.

Yet, the hospital of Saint John in Brussels has not received the attention it deserves in modern scholarship.[51] In the contemporary medieval world, the institution proved to be significant, not only to the people of medieval Brussels, but also to those beyond the city. Jacques de Vitry, for example, numbered Brussels' Saint John hospital among the hospitals of Paris, Noyon, Provins, Tournai and Liège. While the hospitals of Paris, Liège, and Louvain, and others have received specific scholarly attention, a history of the hospital of Saint John is still missing. This proves to be problematic, as many of the institutions in the northern region statutes were modeled on those of the hospital of Saint John, including some named by Jacques de Vitry in his accounts. The hospital of Saint John in Brussels was the model for later hospitals; other hospitals borrowed its statutes and built upon its initial innovations, making it a perfect example of the municipal hospital, as well as the link between medieval charitable institutions and the hospitals we know today.

[51] It should be noted that the lack of attention does not equate to a lack of all scholarship on Saint John hospital. Studies do exist, but they are outdated. Paul Bonenfant's work, from the 1920s to 1965, for example, has helped to bring light to the institution's existence. His efforts included a 1953 cartulary on the hospital. Although an invaluable source, the cartulary is written in French and not readily available to the English-speaking world. Moreover, as a cartulary, it contains 278 charters related to the hospital, but it is not a history of the hospital. Such a history still needs to be deconstructed from the charters of the cartulary, as well as from the extant charters that I have examined within the archives of Brussels. This book, however, is not an updated reassessment of Bonenfant's work; much more can be learned from this remarkable institution. An assessment of the hospital in its social-historical context—that is to say within the development of the medieval town of Brussels, within the growth of the bishopric of Cambrai, and within the increased lay concern for those less fortunate—shows that Saint John was at the center of many developments in medieval Brussels. There, Saint John's became *the* municipal hospital. Extant records from the institution and city archives prove these developments. Other material is drawn from the lives and acts of the bishops of Cambrai, including their mutual training at the University of Paris, the statutes of hospitals both near and afar, and the documentary history of the many peoples involved with the hospital throughout the twelfth and thirteenth centuries.

# PART I

# The History of the Hospital

# CHAPTER 2

# The Hospital in History, c. 3500 BCE–c. 500 CE

**Abstract** This chapter explores the history of the hospital, beginning with early man and ending with Late Antiquity, by providing a brief background as to how certain civilizations—the Egyptians, the Greeks, the Muslims, the Christians, and the Romans—dispensed early healthcare. Key to this chapter is the introduction of temples, the first pseudo hospital, where healing occurred through the supernatural powers of the gods, such as Imhotep and Apollo. "Temple incubation"—as it came to be known—set the stage for later hospital developments, while great medical advancements came with the works of Hippocrates, Galen, Avicenna, and Averroes. Finally, the chapter considers the important public role, or the lack thereof, that governments played in healthcare, as well as the introduction of Christianity.

**Keywords** Egypt · Greece · Rome · Temple incubation · Imhotep · Apollo

## INTRODUCTION

The treatment of the maladies of man is nothing new to the world. Since the beginning of time, disease has plagued mankind and has forced humans—primitive and modern—to search for healing treatments and

© The Author(s) 2018
T. A. Ziegler, *Medieval Healthcare and the Rise of Charitable Institutions*, The New Middle Ages, https://doi.org/10.1007/978-3-030-02056-9_2

cures, the three most basic being washing, bandaging, and producing plasters for setting bones.[1] These remedies may strike one as simple, while the incantations murmured during the process may invoke a notion of primeval witchcraft, sorcery, or even superstition. Too often, though, we are distracted by the oddities of the treatments and strangeness of the words spoken along with them to appreciate just how advanced early man was in terms of healthcare and institutional practices. If, however, we move beyond the seeming absurdities associated with early healthcare, one finds that not only do modern practitioners still employ many of the techniques and use many of the same concoctions, those who performed these skills, from the medicine man to the physician, were highly respected by their community.

Although evidence[2] is scant, paleopathologists have been able to show that early man suffered from disease and sought to eradicate it, thereby creating a need for medicine and care facilities. Many of the medical treatments were simple, as outlined above, and relied on the natural habitat surrounding particular peoples. Plants were steeped in hot water, made into decoctions and plasters, and infused with other herbs to create the first medicines and pharmaceuticals.

Early on, the places of care were limited to homes and public spaces, such as the shared temporary settlements occupied by Paleolithic man

---

[1] Earliest written evidence dates to Mesopotamia and the world's oldest medical document dates from 2100 BCE. It is a partial text of an ancient Sumerian clay tablet that was once buried among the debris at Nippur. For more information, see John L. Webb, "The Oldest Medical Document," *Bulletin of the Medical Library Association*, Vol. 45, No. 1 (January 1957): 1–4. Other ancient texts include the Egyptian Papyri, discussed below.

[2] Evidence comes in a variety of forms, including writing and artistic renderings. Also included as evidence are skeletal remains, which prove to be difficult to discern. For example, one of the more controversial skeletal discoveries is an operation that was performed in the Stone Age was the trephining of skulls. Holes were made in the skull, often successfully, to produce a remedy of some sort. The reasons for why early ancestors used this practice or to what benefit it provided is not clear. The scholarly debate is divided into two camps: supernatural and natural. Paul Broca's work provides the supernatural view that skulls were trephined in order to release "spirits" that caused headaches or even epilepsy. See Paul Broca, "Trépanation chez les Incas," *Bull Acad Méd* (Paris) 32: 866–872; Paul Broca "Sur les Trépanations préhistoriques," *Bull Soc Anthrop* 11: 461–463. Others, such as D. Woelfel, link trepanations to war and weapons, and thus favor a naturalistic view. See D. J. Woelfel, "Die Trepanation" (Anthropos, Bd. 20, 1925). For a more modern view, see Plinio Prioreschi, "Possible Reasons for Neolithic Skull Trephining," *Perspectives in Biology and Medicine*, Vol. 34, No. 2 (Winter 1991): 296–303.

that we today would not consider institutional in nature. The rise of settled territories, governments, bureaucracies, crafts and craftsmen, scientists, and organized religions hastened the development of more advanced treatments and laid the basis for institutional care.

The ad hoc attempts to heal various maladies became more organized as society settled down. While many of the first curatives and practices were certainly rational, the scientific advances of the Neolithic age helped to develop more advanced technologies that allowed the practitioners to better care for their growing societies. Fledging civilizations also began to develop a more formal concept of institutional care. Most patients still received care in the home, but centralized places of treatment, such as the temple, also arose.

The early societies and first civilizations of the Neolithic period had created healthcare systems, which will be defined here as a "local cultural system composed of three overlapping parts: the popular [or non-professional], the professional, and folk sectors."[3] Because a healthcare system is based on a particular local culture, it molded and adapted to the people for whom it served; each society maintained its own treatments, care facilities, and practices. Certain universal norms, however, remained the same, which in turn allows us to make comparisons to modern institutions. We begin our survey in ancient Egypt and continue on to Classical Greece and Imperial Rome before examining healthcare systems in the Middle Ages, as these systems later informed the hospital of the Middle Ages and subsequently, the modern period.[4]

## HEALTHCARE SYSTEMS OF THE 'FIRST CIVILIZATIONS' OF THE FERTILE CRESCENT: EGYPT

The first civilizations of the Fertile Crescent serve as a logical starting point in a survey of western healthcare systems. The cultural uniqueness of ancient Egyptian healthcare, especially in relation to death rituals and

---

[3]Arthur Kleinman, *Patients and Healers in the Context of Culture: An Exploration of the Borderland Between Anthropology, Medicine, and Psychiatry* (Berkeley: University of California Press, 1980), 50. Also, public and private can certainly be substituted for public and private.

[4]Although both Egyptian and Mesopotamian civilizations had active practitioners and healthcare systems, Egypt became the model for the healthcare system adapted by the Greeks and subsequently the Romans, hence the focus on it here.

burial practices, created great advances in medicine and institutional care that served as a standard into the classical period. Egyptian medicinal and institutional practices were later carried to the West, adapted by the Greeks and Romans, and modified in the early Christian periods of Late Antiquity and the Early Middle Ages.

While not intended to be a history of ancient Egypt, a few historical factors need to be explored. Thanks to the many gifts of the Nile River, Egypt eventually grew into a land of villages centralized under the great administration of the pharaoh and his officials, what is often referred to as the pharaonic system. The pharaonic system provided the means for a centralized healthcare system. Agricultural products, taxes, and more were funneled into the capital for the use of the pharaoh to grow his kingdom and power. The pharaoh, believed to be descended of the gods, was equipped with *ma'at*, a system of divinely authorized justice. The ruler's link to the gods, as well as the authority provided to him by the very gods who created him, allowed the pharaoh to claim divine status. The death of a pharaoh, the preparation of his body, and the execution of his burial thus became important in the reunification of the pharaoh with the gods and became a critical component in advanced medicinal care.[5] Moreover, the various capitals of Egyptian bureaucracy became hubs of civilization, supported by the villages that made up the majority of ancient civilization. Governments, artisans, religious officials, scholars, and more were all subsidized under the pharaoh, leading to some of the greatest early advances in science and technology. The two-fold system of technology and pharaonic administration laid the basis for centralized healthcare.[6]

---

[5] For a description of the practices, see Diodorus Siculus, chapter 91–92, 311–317. Diodorus Siculus, *Library of History*, Vol. 1, chapters 91–92, 311–317. *Loeb Classics Online*, http://penelope.uchicago.edu/Thayer/E/Roman/Texts/Diodorus_Siculus/1D*.html.

[6] This is not to say that Egypt was the only ancient civilization to development medical treatments and healthcare systems. Similar accounts existed in Mesopotamia and even Central and South America. The emphasis placed here on Egypt is intentional as in the history of medicine a clear connection can be created from Egypt, to Greece, to Europe in the Middle Ages. India and China also developed sophisticated treatments and centers for care. The religious movement of Buddhism produced a number of hospitals, as Christianity later would. The type of medical treatments first practiced by groups like the Peruvians, the Mesopotamians, and the Egyptians has been termed "archaic medicine" by Owsei Temkin. Temkin argues that although there was progress in medieval treatments and practices, the ancient civilizations of the world still relied on the medicine of the primitives. Moreover,

Much of what we can discern about the professional and nonprofessional, the public and private, aspects of Egyptian healthcare have been preserved in the written records of the Greeks. The Greek historian, Diodorus Siculus, recorded some of the earliest Egyptian practices of care and healing. Diodorus was born in Agyarium, Sicily, and he visited Egypt sometime between 60/59 and 57/56 BCE.[7] The historian began to record his findings in his *Library of History* in 56 BCE. Although far removed from the initial unification of Egypt by Menes, Diodorus' account provides a basis for understanding many of the key components of Egyptian healthcare as they developed throughout the millennia, including diagnoses, treatments, and institutional care.

One of the more interesting aspects recorded is the prevention of illnesses as taken by the Egyptians. Diodorus explains that

> [i]n order to prevent sicknesses they [the Egyptians] look after the health of their bodies by means of drenches, fastings, and emetics, sometimes every day and sometimes at intervals of three or four days. For they say that the larger part of the food taken into the body is superfluous and that it is from this superfluous part that diseases are engendered; consequently the treatment just mentioned, by removing the beginnings of disease, would be most likely to produce health.[8]

Some of these same concepts would be later adopted by the Greeks, especially under Hippocrates, who preferred diet and exercise as a treatment.[9]

Little information is provided regarding public or institutional care; however, Diodorus notes that soldiers "[o]n their military campaigns

"supernaturalism" remained a key component. For more on Owsei Temkin and his ideas, see *A Short History of Medicine*, ed. Erwin H. Ackerknecht and Lisa Haushofer (Baltimore: John Hopkins University Press, 2016), 25–26.

[7] Charles Henry Oldfather, "General Introduction," in Diodorus Siculus, *Library of History*, Vol. 1, No. viii, *Loeb Classics Online*, http://penelope.uchicago.edu/Thayer/E/Roman/Texts/Diodorus_Siculus/1D*.html.

[8] Diodorus Siculus, *Library of History*, Vol. 1, chapter 82, 283, *Loeb Classics Online*, http://penelope.uchicago.edu/Thayer/E/Roman/Texts/Diodorus_Siculus/1D*.html.

[9] "…eating alone will not keep a man well; he must also take exercise. For food and exercise, while possessing opposite qualities, yet work together to produce health." Hippocrates of Cos, *Regimen 1*, 229, *Loeb Classics Online*, https://www.loebclassics.com/view/hippocrates_cos-regimen_i/1931/pb_LCL150.229.xml.

and their journeys in the country [...] all receive treatment without the payment of any private fee," giving credence to the idea that the centralized bureaucracy of the pharaoh's created a pseudo healthcare system. Moreover, we learn that "physicians [drew] their support from public funds and administer[ed] their treatments in accordance with a written law which was composed in ancient times by many famous physicians."[10] Clearly, public funds were set aside to pay for treatments, while physicians were accepted as practitioners of a trade governed by the rules of law.

Like the physicians identified in the Babylonian *Code of Hammurabi* in neighboring Mesopotamia,[11] Egyptian doctors were held accountable, not necessarily for the outcome of the patient but rather the ability to follow the law. According to Diodorus, if a physician obeyed the law as the laws were composed in the sacred book of the "famous ancient physicians," but was unable to save their patient,

> they [were] absolved from any charge and go unpunished; but if they go contrary to the law's prescriptions in any respect, they must submit to a trial with death as the penalty, the lawgiver holding that but few physicians would ever show themselves wiser than the mode of treatment which had been closely followed for a long period and had been originally prescribed by the ablest practitioners.[12]

[10] Diodorus Siculus, *Library of History*, Vol. 1, chapter 82, *Loeb Classics Online*, http://penelope.uchicago.edu/Thayer/E/Roman/Texts/Diodorus_Siculus/1D*.html.

[11] See "Code of Hammurabi," *The Avalon Project*, http://avalon.law.yale.edu/subject_menus/hammenu.asp. It should be noted that the Mesopotamians were also well versed in medical care. Extant evidence survives in the form of medical treatises on cuneiform tablets. The largest of the treatises is the "Treatise of Medical Diagnosis and Prognoses," composed on some forty tablets and dating to c. 1600 BCE. Medical treatment of the individual begins with diagnoses and then cures, starting with the head and ending with the toes. The rational order of prognoses and treatments was accompanied by rational care that parallels modern care. See René Labat, *Traité akkadien de diagnostics et prognostics médicaux* (Academie Internationale d'Historie des Sciences: Paris, 1951). Moreover, it was believed that the Gods created the illnesses, which were diagnosed by an *ashipu*. Important in the diagnosis was identification of which god was causing the illness. The *ashipu* could then administer spells and charms, but for more extensive treatment an *asu*, or physician was needed. See Hector Avalos, *Illness and Health Care in the Ancient Near East: The Role of the Temple in Greece, Mesopotamia, and Israel* (Atlanta: Scholar Press, 1995).

[12] Diodorus Siculus, *Library of History*, Vol. 1, chapter 82, 283, *Loeb Classics Online*, http://penelope.uchicago.edu/Thayer/E/Roman/Texts/Diodorus_Siculus/1D*.html.

The identification of physicians, as well as the laws they were to follow in civil society, indicates the existence of a clearly defined healthcare system that existed in Egypt.

Knowledge of Egyptian healthcare is not limited to outside observers. A large portion of what is known about medical practices in Egypt comes from extant papyri. The bureaucratic nature of the pharaoh's government assured a learned population of scribes, as well as an impetus to record everything from official events to the mundane herbals. The papyri vary in length and completeness—some providing diagnoses and cures and others only diagnoses.[13] Most extant Egyptian records, however, contain remedies, concoctions, and techniques of treatment.

The most remarkable of the surviving papyri include the Edwin Smith Surgical papyrus and the Ebers papyrus.[14] Many cures addressed in the papyri remained simple, while the medical practices of the earliest human societies—washing, bandaging, and plastering—proved essential. The Egyptians, however, expanded their techniques and practices considerably. Among the developments was the concept of the four fundamental elements of earth, water, fire, and air, as well as anatomical knowledge most likely gathered by observation of extensive death rituals and burial practices. In addition, the papyri address a range of specialty topics and techniques, such as dentistry, surgery, and even gynecology. Of special concern were diseases of the stomach (*khet*). The Ebers papyri, for example, discuss ailments of the stomach in the initial paragraphs, in a section on digestion, and in an entire 'book of the stomach'. Diodorus' observation of disease being linked to superfluous and excessive food may help to explain the focus on this particular organ. Other maladies addressed in the papyri include diseases of the head, skin, and heart.[15]

The intimate link between the gods and Egyptian society meant that the gods played a role in healthcare. As identified in the papyri, the gods

---

[13]For more on Egyptian papyri and diagnoses, see J. F. Nunn, *Ancient Egyptian Medicine* (Norman: University of Oklahoma Press, 1996).

[14]The Edwin Smith papyrus was published in 1930 by James Henry Breasted. See John Henry Breasted, *The Edwin Smith Surgical Papyrus* (Chicago: University of Chicago Press, 1930). For more on the Ebers Papyri, see P. W. Bryan, *The Papyrus Ebers* (London: Geoffrey Bles, 1930). Both manuscripts date from the Egyptian Middle Period.

[15]See more on disease in ancient cultures in *Mummies, Disease, and Ancient Cultures*, ed. Aiden and Eve Cockburn (Cambridge University Press: Cambridge, 1980).

were known to have certain remedies to heal themselves.[16] Isis, for example, had a method for healing an illness in Ra's head, which was identified and shared among the practitioners of Egyptian medicine through the papyri.[17] The Egyptians also had a specific god of healing, Imhotep. The historical figure of Imhotep came from a wealthy family, although his status could be considered 'common'. Imhotep was well educated, which allowed him to eventually serve as a vizier to pharaoh Djoser during the third dynasty, c. 2900 BCE. In addition to his official role, Imhotep was also a writer, high priest, scientist, engineer, architect, astronomer, and doctor.[18] His achievements ranged from the building of the stepped pyramid of Djoser to the development of many successful empirical theories of medicine.[19]

Later, in the New Kingdom, beginning c. 1550 BCE, Imhotep became the patron of scribes. His veneration elevated his status, leading eventually to his worship as a god. Imhotep's official deification, c. 525 BCE, designated him as the patron of wisdom and medicine and led to the creation of temples constructed in his honor, which were overseen through the pharaonic bureaucratic system. Although a place worship, the temples incidentally became a place of care, signifying an important transition in healthcare institutions. To be cured of a particular malady, one simply went to the temple and "incubated," or slept. Although this might be perceived as a supernatural practice of healing, it does link together care and institution. In some ways, the first hospital was born.

All in all, Egyptian treatments, care facilities, and practices were clearly in place.[20] From professional to nonprofessional to even folk systems, from public to private, all the components of a healthcare system converged. Although many of the aspects of Egyptian healthcare are straightforward and based on cultural common sense, the systems would be

---

[16] See Bryan, *The Papyrus Ebers*, 45.

[17] Ibid.

[18] Many of these titles come from the Famine Stela where Imhotep is identified. See P. Barguet, *La stèle de la famine à Séhel*, Vol. 34 (Institut français d'archaéologie orientale: Paris, 1953).

[19] The Edwin Smith papyrus has been attributed to Imhotep.

[20] Per Arthur Kleinman's definition, Egypt qualified as having a healthcare system. See above and see Arthur Kleinman, *Patients and Healers in the Context of Culture: An Exploration of the Borderland Between Anthropology, Medicine, and Psychiatry* (Berkeley: University of California Press, 1980), 50.

widely imitated by the Greeks and subsequent followers, namely the connection of religion to medicine and the idea of a place where one could 'incubate' one's illness away. It was simply a matter of time before the practices were adopted and morphed into the hospital of the Middle Ages.

## HEALTHCARE SYSTEMS IN GREECE AND ROME

Imhotep was the father of Egyptian medicine, but he was widely imitated by the Greeks. Although Egypt remained fairly isolated during its early history, the isolation eventually ended as ambitious pharaohs, especially during the New Kingdom, expanded their territories south and east of the Nile Delta. While conquest certainly plays a role in the spreading of ideas and technologies, it is probably more likely that Egyptian medical practices eventually made their way out of the fertile banks of the Nile River through trade. Trade, via both sand routes and sea routes, and especially by groups such as the Phoenicians, carried Egyptian concepts about healthcare to Minoan and Mycenaean Greece and eventually Classical Greece.

While it is difficult to trace the spread of ideas via trade, it is arguably easier to do so by written word. Classical Greece was likely informed of Egypt by writers such as Homer, Herodotus, and Diodorus who visited the foreign land. Thanks to these records we learn, as was the case in Egypt, medical care in Greece was provided through a number of avenues to a variety of people in diverse situations. Homer, for example, discusses wounds in battle in both the *Iliad* and the *Odyssey*. Both epic poems are dated to the eighth century BCE, yet the *Iliad* contains more references to wounds and medicine than the *Odyssey*.[21] Other early evidence for healthcare practices includes the treatment of plague victims in Book One of the *Illiad* to the basic attempts at surgery, especially on the battlefield, while "in the *Iliad* members of certain aristocratic families entered the epic action as experts in the art of healing."[22]

Although most early medical treatments in Greece could be considered common sense applications, later medicinal care, especially in terms of temple gods and incubation, was adopted by the Greeks from Egypt.

[21] R. Hajar, "Learning Ancient Greek Medicine From Homer," *Heart Views*, Vol. 3 (2002): 8.

[22] Timothy S. Miller, *The Birth of the Hospital in the Byzantine Empire* (Baltimore: The Johns Hopkins University Press, 1985, 1997), 31.

According to Diodorus Siculus, Homer,[23] Pythagoras of Samos, Solon the lawgiver, Lycurgus of Sparta, and even the philosopher Plato, visited Egypt. Diodorus argued that these "men[,] who have won the greatest repute in intellectual things[, had] been eager to visit Egypt in order to acquaint themselves with its laws and institutions, which they considered to be worthy of note."[24] The most erudite of scholars studied in Egypt, while their return and the transference of learning was touted, as "all the things for which they were admired among the Greeks were transferred from Egypt."[25]

Herodotus[26] confirms the transmission of various concepts from the Egyptians to the Greeks in Book II of his *Histories*:

> The Egyptians, they said, were the first to discover the solar year, and to portion out its course into twelve parts. They obtained this knowledge from the stars. (To my mind they contrive their year much more cleverly than the Greeks, for these last every other year intercalate a whole month, but the Egyptians, dividing the year into twelve months of thirty days each, add every year a space of five days besides, whereby the circuit of the seasons is made to return with uniformity.)[27]

---

[23] As proof that Homer was in Egypt, Diodous speaks of "evidence, and especially the healing drink which brings forgetfulness of all past evils, which was given by Helen to Telemachus in the home of Menelaüs. For it is manifest that the poet had acquired exact knowledge of the "nepenthic" drug which he says Helen brought from Egyptian Thebes, given her by Polydamna the wife of Thon; for, they allege, even to this day the women of this city use this powerful remedy, and in ancient times, they say, a drug to cure anger and sorrow was discovered exclusively among the women of Diospolis; but Thebes and Diospolis, they add, are the same city." Diodorus Siculus, *Library of* History, Vol. 1, chapter 97, 355, *Loeb Classics Online*, http://penelope.uchicago.edu/Thayer/E/Roman/Texts/Diodorus_Siculus/1D*.html.

[24] Diodorus Siculus, *Library of* History, Vol. 1, chapter 69, 239, *Loeb Classics Online*, http://penelope.uchicago.edu/Thayer/E/Roman/Texts/Diodorus_Siculus/1D*.html.

[25] Diodorus Siculus, *Library of* History, Vol. 1, chapter 96, 327, *Loeb Classics Online*, http://penelope.uchicago.edu/Thayer/E/Roman/Texts/Diodorus_Siculus/1D*.html. Thales even received his medical training in Egypt.

[26] Diodorus preferred the accounts of Homer to those of Herodotus, arguing that Herodotus told "marvelous tales" simply to keep his readers entertained. See Diodorus Siculus, *Library of* History, Vol. 1, chapter 69, 241, *Loeb Classics Online*, http://penelope.uchicago.edu/Thayer/E/Roman/Texts/Diodorus_Siculus/1D*.html. Despite Diodorus' opinion, Herodotus' recordings should not be ignored.

[27] Herodotus, *The History of Herodotus*, Book II, trans. George Rawlinson, Online at http://classics.mit.edu/Herodotus/history.html.

More important is Herodotus' affirmation that the Egyptians "first brought into use the names of the twelve gods, which the Greeks adopted from them; and first erected altars, images, and temples to the gods."[28] Herodotus further stresses that

> my inquiries prove that they were all derived from a foreign source, and my opinion is that Egypt furnished the greater number. For with the exception of Neptune and the Dioscuri, whom I mentioned above, and Juno, Vesta, Themis, the Graces, and the Nereids, the other gods have been known from time immemorial in Egypt. This I assert on the authority of the Egyptians themselves.[29]

He goes on to explain that the gods came first to the Athenians and then later spread to the rest of Greece.[30]

Among the most important of the gods not mentioned above was the Greek god, Apollo, who, if we take Herodotus at his word, was adopted from the Egyptian gods. Apollo, like the Egyptians who had been identified by Diodorus, was the perfect spokesperson for good, holistic, health. He advocated harmony, order, and balance and promoted the idea of "know thy self." Personal discretion of the mind and body was expected: "nothing in excess."[31] Indeed, Apollo's ideas surrounding healthcare were probably borrowed from the Egyptians.

Apollo's importance, however, lay not in his common-sense approaches to good health. Similar to Imhotep, Apollo was the god of healing and known to administer care at his temple through incubation. This idea of temple healing proves key in understanding the transitional developments occurring in healthcare practices. Hector Avalos, for example, has identified that in the Ancient Near East, the temple stood in as a healthcare provider through petition (to the gods), therapy, and thanksgiving.[32] The socio-religious response to the sickness thus became the basis of centralized healthcare: hospitals.

[28] Ibid.

[29] Ibid.

[30] Herodotus, *The History of Herodotus*, Book II, trans. George Rawlinson, Online at http://classics.mit.edu/Herodotus/history.html.

[31] Despite his association with healing, Apollo was also the god of disease and plague.

[32] Avalos demonstrated his arguments in the cases of Greece (especially in connection with the Asclepius—see below), Mesopotamia, and Israel. See Hector Avalos, *Illness and Health Care in the Ancient Near East: The Role of the Temple in Greece, Mesopotamia, and Israel* (Atlanta: Scholar Press, 1995), especially 395, where Avalos discusses the Greek Asclieipion as representative of these three functions.

Apollo was later replaced in the fifth century BCE by the physician, Asclepius, who, according to Greek mythology, was the son of Apollo. Asclepius serves as an important transitional figure between the anthropomorphic god of Apollo and the man, Hippocrates,[33] while his practices, treatments, and places of care represent an evolution to a more permanent healthcare system, including the movement away from supernatural centers of 'incubation' to actual hospitals, or the Asclieipion.[34] These places of care, however, owed their foundation to the early temples and temple healers of Apollo and Imhotep.

Much of what we know about Asclepius and his practices come from anatomical votives used for therapy, petition, and thanksgiving.[35] Asclepius' inventories of anatomical votives in the Athenian Asclieipion included hands, feet, ears, eyes, genitals, wombs, a heart, and a bladder.[36] As 'votives', the items were used in requests for cures or as an offering after as thanks.[37] The votives were then left in the shrines or temples, suggesting that the temple once again served as a locus for healthcare, while the Asclieipion itself was, for all intents and purposes, a hospital.[38] Other Asclepieions were located in Coan, Corinth, and Oropus.[39]

[33] Hippocrates was said to have worshipped Asclepius.

[34] For more on the Asclieipion or Asklepieia, see Miller, *The Birth of the Hospital in the Byzantine Empire*, 38–41. Often associated with Asclepius are his holy staff and snakes, the *caduceus*, which is used to this day to designate medical practitioners and places of care. The *caduceus* may have been a way to inject patients with a non-lethal dose of snake venom, demonstrating an advanced understanding of anti-venoms and medical instruments.

[35] Asclepius was not the only 'god' to have anatomical votives. In fact, "one of the main criteria for characterizing deities as healers is the discovery of pertinent material evidence in the shrines: inscriptions, medical instruments, and funerary and honorary votives with explicit references to illness and healing," in addition to architectural remains and/or literary references. Both Apollo and Asclepius received a large number of votives. See *A Companion to Science, Technology, and Medicine in Ancient Greece and Rome*, Vol. I, ed. Georgia L. Irby (Oxford: Wiley Blackwell, 2016), 442. Moreover, see Hector Avalos for the use of these votives in petition, therapy and thanksgiving in Avalos, *Illness and Health Care in the Ancient Near East: the Role of the Temple in Greece, Mesopotamia, and Israel*.

[36] *A Companion to Science, Technology, and Medicine in Ancient Greece and Rome*, 442.

[37] Ibid.

[38] A school of medicine was located near by.

[39] Peter Barefoot explains that the peoples of the classical world used "locotherapy," be it deliberate or unconscious. Locotheraphy, or attention to environment (earth, water, air, and sun), when building an asklepieion, was key in healing all kinds of maladies. He further argues that the "return to good health is not just a matter of medication or surgery, but the environment must play its part as well." Barefoot argues that some modern hospitals have

The innovations begun under Asclepius were continued by Hippocrates (460–377 BCE). Hippocrates, although best known for the Hippocratic Oath, was significant for the systemization and codification of Greek medicine, much of which is contained in the naturalistic writings of the *Corpus Hippocraticum*.[40] Hippocrates borrowed ideas regarding the four elements of fire, earth, air, and water from early Greek scholars, such as Thales (c. 624–546 BCE) and Pythagoras (c. 570–495 BCE).[41] Later, Greek physicians and philosophers, such as Plato, Aristotle, and Galen, continued the tradition of the four elements, adding to them humors

embraced the idea, but that others would do well to study and adopt the Greek methods. One hospital touted for doing so is Saint Bartholomew's Hospital in London, which has roots in the medieval period. See Peter Barefoot, "Asklepieia: Ideas for Design Today," in *Health and Antiquity*, ed. Helen King (Routledge: New York, 2005), 213–215.

[40] This, of course, contained the *Hippocratic Oath*: "I swear by Apollo Physician and Asclepius and Hygieia and Panaceia and all the gods and goddesses, making them my witnesses, that I will fulfil according to my ability and judgment this oath and this covenant: To hold him who has taught me this art as equal to my parents and to live my life in partnership with him, and if he is in need of money to give him a share of mine, and to regard his offspring as equal to my brothers in male lineage and to teach them this art - if they desire to learn it - without fee and covenant; to give a share of precepts and oral instruction and all the other learning to my sons and to the sons of him who has instructed me and to pupils who have signed the covenant and have taken an oath according to the medical law, but no one else. I will apply dietetic measures for the benefit of the sick according to my ability and judgment; I will keep them from harm and injustice. I will neither give a deadly drug to anybody who asked for it, nor will I make a suggestion to this effect. Similarly I will not give to a woman an abortive remedy. In purity and holiness I will guard my life and my art. I will not use the knife, not even on sufferers from stone, but will withdraw in favor of such men as are engaged in this work. Whatever houses I may visit, I will come for the benefit of the sick, remaining free of all intentional injustice, of all mischief and in particular of sexual relations with both female and male persons, be they free or slaves. What I may see or hear in the course of the treatment or even outside of the treatment in regard to the life of men, which on no account one must spread abroad, I will keep to myself, holding such things shameful to be spoken about. If I fulfil this oath and do not violate it, may it be granted to me to enjoy life and art, being honored with fame among all men for all time to come; if I transgress it and swear falsely, may the opposite of all this be my lot." *The Hippocratic Oath: Text, Translation, and Interpretation*, trans. Ludwig Edelstein (Baltimore: The Johns Hopkins Press, 1943), at http://guides.library.jhu.edu/c.php?g=202502&p=1335752, accessed 4 August 2016. See also, Albert R. Jonson, *A Short History of Medical Ethics* (Oxford: Oxford University Press, 2000), especially chapter 1 on "Hellenic, Hellenistic, and Roman Medicine."

[41] Hakim Mohammed Said, *Traditional Greco-Arabic and Modern Western Medicine: Conflict or Symbiosis?* (Karachi: Hamdard Academy, 1975), 14–15, 20.

(blood, yellow bile, black bile, phlegm) and their respective organs (heart, liver, spleen, and brain).[42] Hippocrates' *Corpus Hippocraticum* serves as the guide to Greek medicine. The focus of the *Copus* is on creating a basic understanding of human physiology. Some of this knowledge was achieved through observation and trial, while other knowledge came from "anatomy," literally the "cutting up" or dissection of the body.[43]

Plato and Aristotle helped to spread the ideas of Hippocrates, but were concerned namely with the philosophical nature of the body, while the medical approaches of Hippocrates and the other Greek physicians was not lost, as Aristotle's pupil, Alexander the Great (356–323 BCE), conquered much of the known world. Alexander, in the wake of his conquests, sought to Hellenize the newly conquered lands, spreading Greek ideas, concepts, building structures, and more throughout the Mediterranean basin, Africa, and Eurasia. This included the creation of Alexandria in Egypt. There, a medical school named the Empirical School was created in 330 BCE and included in its library was the *Corpus Hippocraticum*. Although Alexander's empire was ephemeral, the cultural and intellectual elements of Greece persisted. When the Romans conquered Alexandria in 33 BCE, they helped to transmit Greek medicine and ideas regarding healthcare. Moreover, the spread of Alexander's empire meant the transmission of Greek medicine to Arab, Turkish, and Persian lands. Greek medicine also became highly influential in the later practices of the Muslims.

In the meantime, Roman medicine[44] was slow growing, and rather than a focus being on physicians and temples, Rome, especially during its Empire, focused on public health. We learn of Rome's lack of medicinal care from a legend associated with the Greek temple healer, Asklepios, who was invoked, as the gods had been in the past, to deal with the plague of 295 BCE.[45] Later, the Alexandrine Greek, Asclepiades, "brought literate medicine to Rome around [120 BCE]. He found in sober Rome a folk medicine of myths and simples, administered by the

---

[42] Said, *Traditional Greco-Arabic and Modern Western Medicine: Conflict or Symbiosis?* 17–21.

[43] Ibid.

[44] For more on Roman medicine, see Plinio Prioreschi, *A History of Medicine: Volume III, Roman Medicine* (Omaha: Horatius Press, 1998).

[45] Albert R. Jonsen, *A Short History of Medical Ethics* (Oxford: Oxford University Press, 2000), 9.

*paterfamilias* rather than by physicians."[46] According to one of his successors, Celsus (c. first century BCE to first century CE),[47] Asclepiades helped to "mature our beneficial profession."[48]

Most physicians were drawn from the wealthy classes, while public healthcare projects sought to keep the average Roman citizen clean and healthy. The earliest days of the Roman Republic saw the draining of the marshlands of the seven hills to reduce the spread of diseases like Malaria. This practice continued into the Imperial Age. Innovations such as plumbing, aqueducts, and public baths, constituted one of the more sophisticated healthcare systems of the classical world.

The greatest of the Roman physicians was Galen, or Aelius Galenus, who was born in Pergamum in Asia Minor in 129 CE. Galen later informed Rome of the Greek medical practices. Galen wrote in his *Method of Medicine* that there were five schools of medical thought: dogmatists, rationalists, empiricists, methodics, and pheumatists. Although Galen mostly falls under the dogmatist school, which was also the school of Hippocrates, he did borrow from the other schools as it suited him.[49]

As noted earlier, the Greek hospital, or Asklepieia, was "simply a stoa, or ordinary business arcade, put to nursing use."[50] This plan evolved later into the "Roman *valetudinarium*,[51] or military hospital, [which] was a regular barracks adapted for sick and wounded soldiers."[52] Otherwise, the Romans had temples, while Roman healthcare[53]

---

[46] Jonsen, *A Short History of Medical Ethics*, 9.

[47] For more on Celsus, see Plinio Prioreschi, *A History of Medicine: Volume III, Roman Medicine*, 13.

[48] The text reads *salutaris profession*, which can mean beneficial profession or healing profession. See Jonsen, *A Short History of Medical Ethics*, 9.

[49] Galen, *Method of Medicine*, Books 1–4, ed. and trans. Ian Johnston and G. H. R. Horsley (Cambridge: Harvard University Press, 2011), xlii–xlviii.

[50] John D. Thompson and Grace Goldin, *The Hospital: A Social and Architectural History* (New Haven: Yale University Press, 1975), 5.

[51] For more on the military hospitals, the Valetudinaria, see Miller, *The Birth of the Hospital in the Byzantine Empire*, 38.

[52] For an example of this type of hospital, see the Vindonissa hospital in Windisch, Switzerland, which existed in the first century CE. It is a symmetrical building with a great hall in the middle and patient rooms that lined the corridors. For more information, see Thompson and Goldin, *The Hospital: A Social and Architectural History*, 5. Moreover, Roman hospitals also housed slaves and upper class citizens in their hospitals.

[53] For more on Roman medicine, see Prioreschi, *A History of Medicine: Volume III, Roman Medicine*.

was slow growing with a focus on public health, i.e., baths and aque-ducts. Indeed, "there existed in classical antiquity, [...] little recognition of social responsibility on the part of the individual. Philanthropy among the Greeks [and Romans] did not take the form of private charity, or of a personal concern for those in need, such as orphans, widows, or the sick. There was no religious or ethical impulse for almsgiving. Philanthropic acts were undertaken for the purpose of increasing one's personal reputa-tion."[54] For this reason, healthcare in the Roman Empire was not health-care as much as it was patronage and to some extent philanthropy. Most people would have been cared for through the family, who provided all the basic necessities of life. If sick, a person would have remained in the home, in the sick bed, and a physician, if wealthy enough, would have come to you. Family members, especially women, took care of their own. Otherwise, one might be lucky to find clinics or go to the doc-tor's home, while most care was done at the patient's house. If you were considerably fortunate, you might stumble upon a public physician (*dem-osieuontes iatroi*), who "provided a sophisticated system of free health care, in essence the world's first system of socialized medicine."[55]

Outside of the family and the limited social services, there were few options. Two main options were patronage and philanthropy. Neither was of significant salvation, as they came in the form of money, loans, or doles. In addition, "shelter for the destitute was also far outside the ancient conception of philanthropy."[56] Most people who fell on hard times slept on the streets. There are some wealthy benefactors who endowed education for children, but the concept of charity was not something known to the Romans. Although the establishments created in these early periods might suggest institutionalized municipal care, each group lacked the specific clientele—the poor—and motivations nec-essary for the true municipal hospital, namely those deserving of 'charity' and those giving unselfishly. The rise of Jewish and Christian charities thus became incredibly important for helping the poor and sick.

[54]Gary Ferngren, "The Sick Poor and the Origins of Medical Charity," at http://chreader.org/sick-poor-origins-medical-charity/, accessed 5 October 2017.

[55]Andrew T. Crislip, *From Monastery to Hospital: Christian Monasticism & the Transformation of Health Care in Late Antiquity* (Ann Arbor: University of Michigan Press, 2005), 124. See Cohn-Haft, *Public Physicians*, but his entire argument is based on single piece of evidence from the fifth century CE.

[56]Andrew T. Crislip, *From Monastery to Hospital*, 48.

Initially, and similar to the classical and Jewish, Roman, and Christian civilizations that surrounded them, Arab societies maintained temples for healing. There, priests cared for the sick through prayer and sacrifices, normally to gods associated with healing. Cures, in return, were given by the gods. These practices mimic those of the classical world of the Greeks and Romans, and indeed remained analogous until the sixth and seventh centuries CE. The age of Muhammad (b. 570 CE) ushered in a period that seemed to break with the classical past. Although Allah replaced the gods as the provider of the curative powers,[57] the concept of the temple as a locus of healthcare was abandoned in favor of more secularized centers of care.

Islam was directly linked to the rise of healthcare in the Arab East, as it makes caring for those less fortunate in society a key tenant in the belief system. *The National Library of Medicine* explains that

> in Islam there was generally a moral imperative to treat all the ill regardless of their financial status. The hospitals were largely secular institutions, many of them open to all, male and female, civilian and military, adult and child, rich and poor, Muslims and non-Muslims. They tended to be large, urban structures. The hospital was one of the great achievements of medieval Islamic society. The relation of the design and development of Islamic hospitals to the earlier and contemporaneous poor and sick relief facilities offered by some Christian monasteries has not been fully delineated. Clearly, however, the medieval Islamic hospital was a more elaborate institution with a wider range of functions.[58]

[57] Islamic belief promotes an approach to illness that finds parallels in the ancient world. Just as Apollo was the god of healing and disease, so too is it believed that Allah provides both disease and cures. It is, indeed, only through Allah that disease can be cured: "And if Allah touches you with harm, none can remove it by He, and if He touches you with good, then He is Able to do all things." Surah Al-AnAam, 6: 17 in IqraSense, *Healing and Shifa: From Quran and Sunnah* (USA: IqraSense, 2013), 14. This is very much a spiritual approach to cures. This is not to say that all approaches in Islam were spiritual. Later, a discussion of *The Meadows of Gold* proves the importance placed on scientific cures.

[58] *National Library of Medicine*, "Islamic Culture and the Medical Arts: Hospitals," https://www.nlm.nih.gov/exhibition/islamic_medical/islamic_12.html, accessed 10 August 2016. The early structure of Christianity as a persecuted religion did not allow for such centralized care, while the xenophobic nature of the 'healthcare system' of the Roman Empire was not one to embrace the less fortunate. The transition from the Late Antiquity to the early Middle Ages marked a unique transformation in Christianity, society, culture, and healthcare. The lack of centralization, with the exception of the bureaucracy of the Christian church, made centralized healthcare difficult. As a result, healthcare was overseen by monks and monasteries. Developments that mimicked the Islamic system would have to wait for more urban environments.

Islamic hospitals were multi-functional and served a number of different purposes. Although they were primary centers for medical treatment, they were also used as places of recovery, for mental health patients (asylums), and as retirement homes.[59]

It should thus not come as a surprise that during the Islamic era the Arabian world witnessed a proliferation of hospitals. Often, the title given to the institutions was *Bimaristan*,[60] or the shortened form, *Maristan*.[61] Centralized institutional care was present from as early as the eighth century when Ummayad Caliph Al-Walid I (r. 705–715 CE) founded the first hospice in Jundishapur. Although general care was dispensed, the main mission at the hospice was for the care of lepers. At Jundishapur, Islamic, Persian, and Greek concepts of medicine mixed and merged, while salaried physicians cared for the sick, who largely received care for free.[62] Christian and Jewish physicians may have worked in this and later hospitals, although it is not directly known.[63]

Abbasid Caliph Harun-al-Rashid's (r. 786–809) hospital receives the accolade of the first Islamic hospital.[64] Harun-al-Rashid reigned during a period of great learning, development, trade, luxury, splendor, and economic expansion. His reign included the establishment

---

[59] We will see later that this is paralleled in the hospital of Saint John in Brussels with the exception of the mental health services. Moreover, with the exception of the status of retirement home, most people who sought out care at the hospitals, Islamic and Saint John, were of modest means. The wealthy, in Islamic and Christian societies, would have received care at their homes and/or by court physicians. National Library of Medicine, "Islamic Culture and the Medical Arts: Hospitals," https://www.nlm.nih.gov/exhibition/islamic_medical/islamic_12.html, accessed 10 August 2016.

[60] *Bimaristan* is derived from the Persian word, *birmar*, meaning ill person, while -*stan* denotes place or location, hence place of ill people. *Maristan* is a corrupted form of *bimaristan*. See National Library of Medicine, "Islamic Culture and the Medical Arts: Hospitals," https://www.nlm.nih.gov/exhibition/islamic_medical/islamic_12.html, accessed 10 August 2016.

[61] This was the title that would inform later crusading hospitals in the East.

[62] Jundishapur was also home to a well-known center of learning.

[63] *National Library of Medicine*, "Islamic Culture and the Medical Arts: Hospitals," https://www.nlm.nih.gov/exhibition/islamic_medical/islamic_12.html, accessed 10 August 2016.

[64] The first Christian hospital was founded at the end of the fourth century in Caesaraea in Cappadocia. See Jonsen, *A Short History of Medical Ethics*, 13.

of the Bayt al-Hikma, or the House of Wisdom. In addition, Harun-al-Rashid had social compassion and sought to care for those less fortunate, as best illustrated in *The Meadows of Gold*.[65] During the Islamic Golden Age, Caliph Harun-al-Rashid had his vizier, Yahya, and built the first *bimaristan* in Baghdad. The hospital was headed by Harun's personal physician, Jibrial Bakhtishu (d. c. 828–829). Jibrial attended the Persian (Sasanid) academy of Gundeshipur (Jundishapur), where the first Islamic leprosarium had been created. The success of the first *bimaristan* encouraged the building of several more hospitals in Baghdad and throughout the Islamic World, and as a result, Christians would later come into contact with the *birmaristans* in their expeditions to the east.[66]

At each juncture, from Egypt to Greece to Rome to the Islamic world, developments were made in healthcare practices and treatments and in the creation of institutionalized care. The temples of the ancient and classical world evolved into the hospitals of the urban Islamic world. Centralized care became more apparent as time went on. What largely influenced the development of the medieval hospital, though, was yet to come: Christianity.

---

[65] There are a number of sections that can be highlighted in this work, but key is a section titled, "Wathqid Discusses Medicine," which details Islamic practices in medicine. See Masudi, *The Meadows of Gold*, ed. and trans. Paul Lunde and Caroline Stone (New York: Routledge, 2010).

[66] There is a direct connection between the birmaristans of the Middle East, and particularly of Jerusalem, to Brussels and the Hospital of Saint John. Those hospital connections help to create a link that solidifies transference of the idea of centralized care overseen by a governmental—albeit religious in some sense—from the East to the West. With the hospital of Saint John, that very transition occurred; it was initiated by Duke Godfrey but augmented by trade and civic centers, such as Brussels, which was located on a primary east–west trade route. Brussels was a second-generation Roman city that lost much of its Roman influence with the decline of the Empire. The shrinking of Roman Imperial and pagan influence meant the replacement with Christian institutions. The cities were reorganized—topography shifted to that of the church. It will be illustrated later that in Brussels, the dukes of Brabant and the Bishops of Cambrai, in addition to the city aldermen, vied for control as the socio/politico/religio leaders. This is evident in the rise of the hospital of Saint John, which again was borrowed largely from the East.

## THE INFLUENCE OF CHRISTIANITY

The municipal hospital as we understand it today developed thanks to a unique combination of concepts, beginning in the waning periods of the Roman Empire with the birth of Christianity. Christianity brought a focus on charity: *caritas*.[67] For Christians, charity, healthcare, and the poor were inextricably linked, while care for the poor and sick became a necessary condition of Christian salvation.[68] Charity, in addition, would provide the foundation for the early *hospes*, or hospital, as "the sick person in Greco-Roman antiquity was "less than fully a human being.""[69] As one medical historian writes describing Greco-Roman society: "The sick man, the cripple, the weakling are less worthwhile men and can only be reckoned as such in the view of society. Their worth is determined solely in terms of the possibility for bettering their condition. A lifetime of sickness was completely despised. Antiquity offers no evidence of any provision for the care of the crippled. A sick man must become well again in order to count again as a worthwhile person."[70] Thus, in the Greco-Roman times, the sick lived on the margins of society because they lacked a defined role within that society.[71] The exception to this came with Jewish and Christian charity and later with monasticism.

As noted in the introduction, *caritas* was defined first as "dearness, costliness, high price" in association with objects that were highly valued.[72] The definition evolved to include "regard, esteem, affection,

---

[67] This is not to say that peoples other than the Christians did not practice charity. As noted earlier, the Romans understood that clean and healthy citizens were happy citizens. Charity was, in fact, a central tenant of Islam as well.

[68] Mollat, *The Poor in the Middle Ages*, 38.

[69] Darrel Amundesen and Gary Ferngren, "Medicine and Religion: Pre-Christian Antiquity," in *Health/Medicine in the Faith Traditions*, ed. Martin Marty (Philadelphia: Fortress Press, 1982), 88 in Andrew T. Crislip, *From Monastery to Hospital: Christian Monasticism & the Transformation of Health Care in Late Antiquity* (Ann Arbor: University of Michigan Press, 2005), 69.

[70] Henry E. Sigerist, "The Special Position of the Sick," in *Culture, Disease, and Healing*, ed. David Landry (New York: Macmillan, 1977), 388–394, at 391 in Andrew T. Crislip, *From Monastery to Hospital: Christian Monasticism & the Transformation of Health Care in Late Antiquity* (Ann Arbor: University of Michigan Press, 2005), 69.

[71] Andrew T. Crislip, *From Monastery to Hospital*, 69.

[72] *A Latin Dictionary*, "*caritas*," ed. Charlton Lewis and Charles Short (The Clarendon Press: Oxford University Press, 1962), 292. See use, for example, by Cicero and Cato.

[and] love" in a more brotherly sense,[73] while *caritates* were "the loved persons."[74] In short, it can mean both love and charity.[75] In a more modern sense, charity takes on the idea of caring for those who do not have the means or wherewithal to care for themselves, whereas in the early history of the first millennium, charity encompassed healthcare and care for the sick. The provision of healthcare and generalized care for the poor in early Christianity is but one component of *caritas*; yet, it was the component that not only set the Christians apart from their Classical counterparts, but also helped to define what healthcare would become in the later Roman Empire and the early Middle Ages.

Many notions on how to provide healthcare and how to care for the sick in early Christian communities were derived from interpretations of James 5:14–15 in the Christian New Testament.[76] If a person is sick and desires to be healed, the elders of the church are called upon to pray the prayer of faith: "the prayer of the faith will save the sick, and the Lord shall raise them up, and if sins they may have committed, they shall be forgiven to him."[77] Christians are then to confess their sins "to one another, and pray for one another, so that [they] may be healed."[78] This practice bears a striking similarity to the Greco-Roman temple incubation and votive offerings, yet the temple and ritual have been replaced with the Christian church and prayer.[79]

[73] Lewis and Short, 292.

[74] Ibid.

[75] Peter Kwaniewski explains that *caritas* should be translated as "charity;" he argues, "the fact that for some people "charity" has come to mean nothing other than tossing a coin into a beggar's cup is no reason to throw it out of theology where it occupies the queenliest of places; like many another beautiful but endangered species in the English language, it rather needs to be rescued and bred in captivity. For the scholastics, charity means nothing less than the very love which is God's essence, the love that Christ manifested in his death on the cross." Things like almsgiving are what Kwaniewski calls "charity's effects." See Peter Kwaniewski, in Thomas Aquinas, *On Love and Charity: Readings from the Commentary on the Sentences of Peter Lombard*, trans. Peter A. Kwaniewski, Thomas Bolin, and Joseph Bolin (Washington, DC: The Catholic University Press of America, 2008), xxii.

[76] See Frederick S. Paxton, *Christianizing Death: The Creation of a Ritual Process in Early Medieval Europe* (Cornell University Press, 1996), 27.

[77] James 5:14–15, RSV.

[78] James 5:16, RSV.

[79] The passage in James, however, like many in the Christian Bible, has multiple meanings, including both the literal prayer for healing the more spiritual idea that sickness, or sin, can be healed through prayer. Contextually, because James is not necessarily 'sick'

The discussion in James of the anointing of the sick serves as a key component to understanding healthcare in the bible and within early Christian communities, while both the life of Jesus Christ and the deeds of his twelve apostles become models for how to care for the sick. Christians, for example, took to heart Jesus' Sermon on the Mount, "Blessed of are the poor...,"[80] as well as the idea that those who had provided care would find eternal salvation: "I was sick and you took care of me."[81] Jesus himself was a healer: "News about Him spread all over Syria, and people brought to Him all who were ill with various diseases, those suffering acute pain, the demon-possessed, those having seizures, and the paralyzed–and He healed them."[82] A similar passage is found in Mark 6:13 when the twelve apostles "drove out many demons **and** (sic.) anointed many sick people with oil and healed them."[83] Finally, charity and caring for the sick served to fulfill aspects of the seven corporal works of mercy, which also included feeding the hungry, giving drink to the thirsty, welcoming the stranger, clothing the naked, visiting the sick, visiting the prisoner, and burying the dead.[84] To gain the favor of Christ on the Day of Judgment, Christians were enjoined to care for the sick.[85]

but instead is fighting a spiritual battle, it is more likely that this passage is associated with spiritual healing. A similar situation occurs in Islam. Although there is an idea linked to physical care, belief and faith become components for true spiritual healing, or *ruqyah*: "And We send down of the Quran that which is healing and a mercy to those who believe." Quran, Surah Al-Israa, 17:82 in IqraSense, *Healing and Shifa: From Quran and Sunnah* (USA: IqraSense, 2013), 20.

[80] Matthew 5:3, RSV.

[81] Matthew 25:36, RSV.

[82] Matthew 4:24, RSV.

[83] It is my interpretation that there are two different actions occurring: one is the casting out of demons and the other is the healing of the sick by anointing them. Most Greek versions of the text suggest a break in the two actions with a comma. This is seen in Scrivener's Textus Receptus of 1894: "καὶ δαιμόνια πολλὰ ἐξέβαλλον, (sic.) καὶ ἤλειφον ἐλαίῳ πολλοὺς ἀρρώστους καὶ ἐθεράπευον." The Stephanus Textus Receptus of 1550, however, does not have the delineation between the two actions: "καὶ δαιμόνια πολλὰ ἐξέβαλλον καὶ ἤλειφον ἐλαίῳ πολλοὺς ἀρρώστους καὶ ἐθεράπευον." For Greek translations, see http://biblehub.com/texts/mark/6-13.htm.

[84] These ideas are based on Matthew 25:31–46 RSV, where Matthew lists the six virtues that Jesus will use on the Day of Judgment: "I was sick and you took care of me," etc. To these six was added Tobit 1:17–19 RSV, which includes the burying of the dead. It is no coincidence that medieval monks practiced the seven corporal works of mercy. The monastery became a pseudo hospital for the sick in the Middle Ages. See below for more information.

[85] Andrew T. Crislip, *From Monastery to Hospital*, 54.

Some of what we know about care for the sick in early Christianity comes from Dionysius, bishop of Alexandria from 247 to 264 CE. Dionysius wrote,

> the most, at all events, of our brethren in their exceeding love and affection for the brotherhood were unsparing of themselves and clave to one another, visiting the sick without a through as to the danger, assiduously ministering to them, tending them in Christ, and so most gladly departed this life along with them; being infected with the disease from others, drawing upon themselves the sickness from their neighbors, and willingly taking over their pains. And many, when they had cared for and restore to health others, died themselves, thus transferring their death to themselves.[86]

The key in the visitation was caring for those who did not have the family to do so. This set a precedent in the ancient world of care for all that continued on to the Middle Ages, and it was uniquely Christian as compared to Roman. Christian churches also provided for those without family and means.

This all-encompassing care was at the heart of healthcare. As noted in the introduction, healthcare is a blanket term for the care of individuals via diagnosis and treatment.[87] Healthcare seeks to improve physical and mental conditions, illnesses, diseases, and injuries, while healthcare professionals, such as physicians, nurses, dentists, midwifes, pharmacists, and more all play key roles in the delivery of various treatments. Treatments range for medicinal (i.e., medical care or professional treatment as dictated by the guidelines of the professional medical community), to herbal, to therapeutic, and beyond. Healthcare in the modern world tends to be an all-encompassing approach to the well-being of an individual. Remove the birth of 'modern medicine' after the scientific revolution, and the definition becomes the characterization of healthcare in the late Roman Empire and early Middle Ages, thanks to Christianity and concepts of *caritas*.

Overall, charity, at least in the form of caring for the sick and poor, grew out of the life and actions of Jesus Christ  and his apostles. The ideas put forth in the first years of the millennium regarding Christian

---

[86] Andrew T. Crislip, *From Monastery to Hospital*, 55. For more from Dionysius, see Eusebius.

[87] Sometimes, prevention is also included as an element of healthcare.

*caritas* were carried on by Christians and developed into more sophisticated forms of healthcare, especially as the organization of the church increased, which will be explored momentarily. It should be noted first, though, that the idea of caring for someone in need was not new to monotheistic Abrahamic religions. The Jewish synagogue, for example, served as a meeting place, a community center, a religious hub, a location for social activities, education, prayers, meetings, and charity.[88] Of these many elements, one of the most important for the Jewish community was the focus on charity through the creation of "community agencies for feeding the poor, clothing the needy, caring for the sick, burying the dead, ransoming captives, educating orphans, and providing poor girls with dowries."[89]

The Jewish traditions[90] persisted in early Christian communities as "clubs,"[91] which can be seen in the writing of the early Church Father, Quintus Septimius Florens Tertullianus c. 155–230 CE (Tertullian).[92] According to Tertullian, Christians maintained "clubs," the predecessor of the Jewish clubs and the precursor of the later confraternities. The club is described in his *Apology* as "an association (*corpus*) based on shared religious conviction, the unity of [the Christian] way of life, and the bond of common hope."[93] Tertullian included care for the poor and/or sick as one of the defining components of Christian clubs, and he

---

[88] Everett Ferguson, *Backgrounds of Early Christianity* (Grand Rapids: William B. Eerdmans, 1993), 540.

[89] Everett Ferguson, *Backgrounds of Early Christianity*, 540.

[90] There is a distinction, however, in how the two groups—Christians and Jews—approached care of the sick. According to Luke 13:10–17, for example, the chief rabbi of the synagogue criticizes Jesus for healing a woman. This issue is not in the care that he gives or she receives, but in the fact that he performed the act on the Sabbath. See Miller, *The Birth of the Hospital in the Byzantine Empire*, xvii. For more on Jewish charity, see Frank M. Loewenberg, *From Charity to Social Justice* (New Brunswick: Transaction Publishers, 2001); Gildas Hamel, *Poverty and Charity in Roman Palestine: First Three Centuries, C.E.*, Near Eastern Studies 23 (Berkeley: University of California Press, 1990).

[91] There are even some modern arguments that Imhotep of Egypt was the biblical Joseph, which is key in making the connections between temple incubation and early hospitals.

[92] Quintus Septimius Florens Tertullianus was born in and probably spent the majority of his life in Carthage—a Phoenician settlement.

[93] Tertullian, *Apology* 39.1–6, in A. D. Lee, *Pagans and Christians in Late Antiquity: A Sourcebook* (New York: Routledge, 2000), 37–38.

praised the Christian "clubs" for caring for the poor, for providing burial, and for giving homes to orphans.[94]

Christian practices toward the poor and sick, the mixing of Roman and Jewish traditions, and the basic tenets of Christian belief vis-à-vis the Christian bible, the life of Jesus Christ, and the actions of the twelve apostles, all grew to encourage philanthropy and charity in the fledgling church of the Roman Empire. As the early church began to grow, so too did church organization that included provisions for healthcare. Charity became the responsibility of the church deacon, who was responsible for dispensing money and goods. Thus, it was the deacon who was to provide hospice to pilgrims and care for the sick.[95]

Hippolytus (c. 215 CE), in chapter thirty-four of his *Apostolic Tradition*, explains the role of the subdeacons and bishops. Subdeacons and deacons are to report to the bishop those "who are sick." If the bishop wishes, "he may visit them." Hippolytus goes on to note that "the sick man is much comforted that the high priest remembered him,"[96] once again invoking that idea of god-like visitation seen in Egyptian, Greek, and Roman cultures. Beyond visiting the sick, bishops were also required to teach charity. Finally, Hippolytus identifies in his work the equivalent to the modern prebend, who was placed in charge of caring for the poor.[97] The creation of the prebend was an important step in the transition to the hospitals of the Middle Ages. The prebendary, or revenues that supported charity, helped to put in place an organized system of care within the Christian jurisdictional organization. Later, prebendaries were often synonymous with hospital masters.

The idea, however, of a specialized hospital under the supervision of a prebendary would take time to develop, and because of the amalgamation with concepts of Christian charity, Christian hospitals would

---

[94] The Christian clubs were significantly different from Roman clubs and associations. Roman clubs included three types: economic (*stationes*), religious (*cultores*) and social (*tenuiores*). All three types had some sort of religious function, but paled in comparison to their Christian counterparts. Some emperors tolerated the associations while others called for their disbandment.

[95] Carter Lindberg, *Love: A Brief History Through Western Christianity* (Oxford: Blackwell, 2008); Carter Lindberg, *Beyond Charity: Reformation Initiatives for the Poor* (Minneapolis: Fortress Press, 1993), 44.

[96] Hippolytus, *The Apostolic Tradition of Hippolytus*, ed. Gregory Dix (London: SPCK, 1968), 57.

[97] Mollat, *The Poor in the Middle Ages*, 40.

normally be attached to other Christian associations, such as the clubs identified above and later in association with monasteries. In examining the meanings and definitions of the word "hospital" one finds several derivatives. One meaning of the term is taken from the word *hospes*, meaning simply a host or guest,[98] whereas houses for wayfarers and the sick were sometimes simply called "houses of hospitality."[99] In another view, "the word *hospital* comes from the Greek word *hospitum*, a word that is mentioned frequently in the literature from the fifth century CE onward."[100]

"Hospital" and "houses of hospitality" differ greatly from the first healing building discussed: the Greek Asklepieia. Early Christian hospices and hospitals, however, took on more of a monastic form,[101] conforming to the idea of houses of hospitality. The early 'houses of hospitality' were initially for pilgrims and only later saw to the sick.[102] By the fourth century and the Council of Nicaea (325 CE), the formal process of setting up hospitals was well under way.[103]

Canon LXX of the Council required a hospital to be set up in every cathedral city, largely because cathedral cities attracted pilgrims, many of whom arrived ill. Moreover, Canon LXX specified that "if the goods of the hospital are not sufficient for its expenses he [the hospital superintendent] out to collect all the time and from all Christians provision

[98] Clay, *The Medieval Hospitals of England*, 1.

[99] Ibid.

[100] Donald Snook, Jr., *Hospitals: What They Are and How They Work* (Maryland: Aspen Publishers, 1992), 3.

[101] For example, see Turmanin in Syria (on the main road from Antioch to Qalat-Siman) (475 CE)—it was built over the pillar upon which St. Simeon Stylites dwelled. See Thompson and Goldin, *The Hospital: A Social and Architectural History*, 7.

[102] There is not as great of a distinction between a pilgrim and a sick person as one might first believe. Thompson and Goldin note that "the definition of a pilgrim is more or less sick, he or she having undertaken a long journey as a form of penance." Travel was difficult for people, both physically and mentally. There was a general need for nurses to care for and bandage feet from the roads. Thus, "for this reason the convent shelter [had to] be more than an inn, nursing care would necessarily be included in hospitality, and a hospice had to be part hospital." See Thompson and Goldin, *The Hospital: A Social and Architectural History*, 7–8. Never is this truer than in the Christian Crusades of the eleventh and twelfth centuries. The establishment of the crusader hospitals, and even the order of the Hospitallers, is a combination of the house of hospitality and the more military-esque hospital of the Egyptians, Greeks, and Romans.

[103] Thompson and Goldin, *The Hospital: A Social and Architectural History*, 3–4.

according to the ability of each."[104] The alms were then used "as a public service and [to establish] hospitals, already devoted to particular specialties, in cities and along major roads."[105] A short time later, the first Christian hospital was founded at the end of the fourth century in Caesarea in Cappadocia.[106] Most of these hospitals would decline with the fall of the Empire, giving way to predominantly monastic institutions.

Overall, the arrival of Christianity to the Roman Empire marked a distinct change in the approach to healthcare. Traditionally, the poor died on the streets of the Roman Empire.[107] Beyond efforts of civic improvement, there was little done to help the poor and sick. This is principally because the world of Rome knew no division between rich and poor; rather, the distinction was between the citizen and the non-citizen.[108] This created an environment where the "benefactors of cities gave to their "fellow citizens" and never to the poor. [...] They received entertainment, public comforts (such as great bathhouses), and (in many cities) considerable dole of food."[109] What they did not receive was healthcare, at least not in the Christian sense.

Roman Law originally separated the classes into patrician and plebian and dictated that no intermarriage should take place between the two. The love that the patricians had was for their city, not their people. There was no such thing as charity in the Roman Republic or Empire. Christianity, however, changes this, as evident in the revision to

---

[104] Documents from the First Council of Nicea [The First Ecumenical Council], Henry R. Percival, ed., *The Seven Ecumenical Councils of the Undivided Church*, Vol XIV of Nicene and Post Nicene Fathers, 2nd series, ed. Philip Schaff and Henry Wace (repr. Edinburgh: T&T Clark; Grand Rapids MI: Wm.B. Eerdmans, 1988). *Fordham Internet Sourcebook*, at http://sourcebooks.fordham.edu/halsall/basis/nicea1.txt, accessed 15 August 2016.

[105] Mollat, *The Poor in the Middle Ages: An Essay in Social History*, 19–20. This notion about the establishment of hospitals along roads is paramount when considering some of the developments highlighted in the previous chapter. Brussels arose along old Roman trade routes, and many of the cultural remnants of the new city were Roman in origin. The fact that Brussels came to embody so many hospitals in its medieval apex should not be a surprise given the fact that most hospitals formed along roads and in major cities.

[106] See Jonsen, *A Short History of Medical Ethics*, 13.

[107] Thompson and Goldin, *The Hospital: A Social and Architectural History*, 4–6.

[108] Peter Brown, *Through the Eye of a Needle: Wealth, the Fall of Rome, and the Making of Christianity in the West 350–550 AD* (Princeton: Princeton University Press, 2014), 68.

[109] Brown, *Through the Eye of a Needle*, 68.

Roman Law under Theodosius II (*Codex Theodosianus*, 429 CE), which decreed that "the peoples who are ruled by the administration of Our Clemency shall practice that religion which the divine Peter Apostle transmitted to the Romans."[110] The revisions to the law instituted and required care for the poor: "the poor must be supported by the wealth of the churches."[111] Clergy, now favored under Roman law, were to care for the poor and sick. This helps to set up the transition from a lack of healthcare in the Roman Empire to the emerging systems of healthcare in the early Middle Ages, as largely overseen by monasteries.

Moreover, the Christian tenet of giving to the poor and caring for the sick was not part of the Roman vocabulary. The Roman elite were wired to give to citizens, but not to the poor.[112] Convincing Roman populations to give to the poor would mean a complete change in societal norms, moving the plebian citizen down the social ladder into the category of poor. As a result, the "classical view of society as made up of a honey-comb of civic groups was replaced, across Europe, by the gray and universal vision of a world divided only between the rich and poor."[113] The evolution provoked changes to society, to city structure, and to healthcare; a new emphasis was placed on the "the otherworldly efficacy of pious gifts both to the poor and to the church."[114] These evolutions were incredibly important in the transition to the Middle Ages, as the type of healthcare that emerged was unique in many ways from its Greco-Roman predecessors. The distinctive type of healthcare that would arise in the early Middle Ages would eventually find its apogee in the high medieval hospital.

## CONCLUSION

The development of healthcare systems in the west was slow going, but at each juncture, serious advances occurred. The earliest groups of people focused on the basic healing techniques of washing, bandaging, and plastering. Greater developments emerged with the Egyptians, whose centralized bureaucratic system allowed medicinal practices to advance

---

[110] *The Theodosian Code and Novels and the Sirmondian Constitutions*, trans. Clyde Pharr (Princeton: Princeton University Press, 1980), 440–451.

[111] *The Theodosian Code and Novels and the Sirmondian Constitutions*, 440–451.

[112] Brown, *Through the Eye of a Needle*, 68.

[113] Brown, *Through the Eye of a Needle*, 70–71.

[114] Brown, *Through the Eye of a Needle*, 71.

more rapidly. The progress in Egypt included the rise of a basic health-care system made up of the three-fold professional, nonprofessional, and folk sectors, while the socio-religious culture created an early hospital-like institution through temple incubation. These concepts were widely imitated by the Greeks, borrowed by the Romans, improved upon by the Byzantines, to be explored next chapter, and adapted by the Christians. The introduction of Christianity, however, saw the rise of several new issues, namely the concept of *caritas*. To care for the sick was no longer something limited to the governmental administration; it was now the duty of every Christian citizen patrician and plebian alike.

With the decline of the Roman Empire, organized civic healthcare dwindled and passed to some of the only institutions still available for such care: the monastery. The monastery would be the main provider of healthcare through out the early Middle Ages. The high Middle Ages, however, saw the rise of towns and a revived combination of Christian service and civic awareness that was not achieved in late antiquity and the early Middle Ages because of the political decentralization and the lack of cities. It was a revival of the "honeycomb of civic groups"[115] that had once ruled the Roman Empire; it was a revival of the "institutionalized groups—benefactors, town councilors, and *populus*"[116] who had once made Rome. Combined with factors, such as the rise of trade and the influence of Islamic medicine, it was the basis for the first municipal hospital.

[115] Ibid.
[116] Brown, *Through the Eye of a Needle*, 70.

# CHAPTER 3

# Early Medieval Charitable Institutions and Hospitals, c. 500–1000 CE

**Abstract** The decline of the Roman Empire signaled many changes for Western Europe, including the evolution of the early medieval hospital. Prior to the early Middle Ages, hospitals and healthcare were the responsibility of governments and private individuals. A lack of stabilizing forces c. 500 CE obliged others to provide healthcare. Christians, and especially monasteries, took up the reins; the concern that Christians had for those less fortunate merged with the Roman notion of *Amor civicus*, love for one's city. The end of the early Middle Ages witnessed a major change as new concepts of healthcare, from Byzantium, and medical treatises, especially from the Islamic world, made their way into Italy, setting the stage for an explosion of lay hospitals in the next two hundred years.

**Keywords** *Amor civicus* · Monasteries · Basileias · Byzantium · *Regula* · *Caritas*

The rise of what might be titled the early medieval hospital was anything but subtle. The chaos that engulfed the Western Roman Empire in the fourth and fifth centuries forced citizens and foreigners alike to develop substitutes for the declining administrative structure that was once overseen by imperial figures. Groups, such as the Catholic Church and its leadership via the papacy, various barbarian leaders, and

© The Author(s) 2018

T. A. Ziegler, *Medieval Healthcare and the Rise of Charitable Institutions*, The New Middle Ages, https://doi.org/10.1007/978-3-030-02056-9_3

even monasteries, emerged as stabilizing powers in the wake of declining governmental agencies. The rise of the church, the decline of the Empire, and the concept of *caritas* allowed for the eventual emergence of the monastic hospital, a major step toward the high medieval municipal hospital. Moreover, the rise of a gift-giving society led to the creation of lay-funded and founded hospitals, the precursor to the high medieval municipal hospital, while advances in medical practices paved the way for the developments of the high Middle Ages.

## THE HOSPITALS OF LATE ANTIQUITY AND THE EARLY MIDDLE AGES

As the Later Roman Empire continued to merge with Christianity, imperial authorities and the church officials cooperated in efforts of civic well-being and healthcare. As had commonly been the case, the pride the Roman citizen had for his city was immense. Peter Brown argues that the "phenomenon of civic euergetism [was] widespread in the Greco-Roman world" and its manifestations "vivid," giving credence to the phrase "*Amor civicus*. Love of the city."[1] Evidentiary proof lies in the Roman "temples, the forums and public buildings, the arches, the colonnades, and the vast places of public entertainment."[2] This idea of love for one's city did not go away with the invasions and political decentralization of the fourth and fifth centuries, but it did transform.

Rather than public buildings for entertainment and indulgence, the need instead turned to the people and the places of care, thanks largely to the concept of *caritas*. Moreover, declining power in the West, the lack of an effective military force, and the persistence of Germanic tribes along the Roman frontier created a power vacuum. As a result, church leaders found themselves increasingly filling leadership roles and thus became responsible for civic creations.[3] For example, Bishop Deogratias

---

[1] Brown, *Through the Eye of a Needle*, 63.

[2] Brown, *Through the Eye of a Needle*, 64.

[3] Men and women, lay and religious alike, contributed to the growing tradition—*Amor civicus* was not limited to church figures alone. While some early hospitals were available to the masses, those who wished to receive care at home relied on women. For example, even early in the history of Christian healthcare, "the Roman aristocrat Fabiola, praised by Jerome, showed her Christian devotion by founding a hospital and nursing in it." See Gillian Clark, *Women in Late Antiquity: Pagan and Christian Life-Styles* (Oxford: Clarendon Press, 1993), 68.

of Carthage (d. 457), who ransomed church possessions in 439 in order to free captives taken by the Vandals, was one such figure who helped to fill that void.[4] Deogratias also arranged for two churches, the Basilica Fausti and the Basilica Novarum, to be used to house displaced persons. In many ways, the bishop became the new father of the poor.

In other places, bishops simply set up charitable institutions and hospitals. Bishop Masona (d. c. 600/610) managed to bring public healthcare to Visigothic Spain. He "established many monasteries, enriching them with much land, he built several churches of marvelous construction, and he brought many souls to dedication to God there."[5] He also "built a hospice (*xenodocium*) [580] and endowed it with great estates, and after providing it with servants and doctors, he commanded them to devote themselves to the needs of travelers and the sick."[6] Masona then used the money from the land to develop the hospital and staff doctors. There, most care was given to travelers and pilgrims, the primary recipients of healthcare throughout the Middle Ages.

Although attempts such as these at civic welfare were present, they should not been seen as centralized; political decentralization disrupted any orderly development of healthcare. As a result, much of the effort to provide poor relief and healthcare fell to the "friends of God,"[7] especially monks, while the majority of care was overseen by monks in the "houses of hospitality." For monks, philanthropy was at the heart of their vows; monks were "obsessed"[8] with healthcare, which incidentally allowed

[4] Victor of Vita, *History of the Persecution of the Province of Africa*, "The Charity of Deogratias, Bishop of Carthage, to the Captives Brought from Rome by the Vandals," 1.24–6 in *Readings in Late Antiquity: A Sourcebook*, ed. Michael Maas (New York: Routledge, 2000), 311–312.

[5] "Episcopal organization of charitable institutions," 12.10, *Lives of the Holy Fathers of Merida*, 5.3 in *Pagans and Christians in Late Antiquity: A Sourcebook*, ed. A. D. Lee (New York: Routledge Press, 2000), 225–226.

[6] Ibid.

[7] This term is borrowed from Peter Brown. See Peter Brown, *The Making of Late Antiquity* (Cambridge: Harvard University Press, 1978), especially chapter 3.

[8] Crislip, *From Monastery to Hospital*, 39. "Early monastic leaders obsessed over sickness and health. A deep concern with illness runs through all early monastic literature, the lives, rules, instructions, and homilies." It should be noted that at the monastic hospital, the main concern was for the soul, yet, patients were given basic treatments, including those most employed by the earliest of peoples: cleaning, bandaging, and plastering/setting bones. Herbal remedies were provided and prayers, or invocations to Christ, were said. For herbal remedies, see, for example, the works of Matthew Platearius, *Circa instans*. Matthew was the chief authority on pharmaceutical ingredients, or *material medica*. His

"monastic leaders [to] develop systems from providing health care to all monastics and incorporate all manner of sick and disabled individuals into monastic society."[9] The key word in this sentence is *all*; there was no limit for whom care was provided. The transition to providing for all—for those who did not take vows—was, however, a lengthy process.

As beautifully noted by Andrew T. Crislip, "monasticism influenced virtually all areas of the late antique world. [...] [M]onasticism also transformed the healthcare system of Late Antiquity."[10] The question becomes why; why did monks gravitate toward healthcare? The simple answer is that monks had to deal with both sickness and health within the monastery. For the monastic, you renounced all ties to secular life; you could no longer rely on family support, so you needed the monastery hospital.[11] The monastery hospital was designed first to care for monastic members of the monastic family. It provided food, clothing, shelter, and of course, healthcare.

Once those ideas were coupled with Christian ideas of *caritas*, it was a logical step for monastic leaders to focus "on problems of the establishment of a healthcare system and the creation of a positive social role for the sick within monastery life."[12] The merging of monastic life and the social need provided via *caritas* led to a protohospital complete with professional nurses and an infirmary. This process was revolutionary. For the first time historically speaking, we see a destigmatization of healthcare[13] and the rise of the true hospital. The timing was perfect, in that the control of hospital through monastic social services "was subordinated to

---

work survives in hundreds of extant copies in Latin and many other translated into a variety of European languages. Matthew Platearus, *Circa instans*, in *Medieval Italy: Texts in Translation*, 316–321.

[9] Crislip, *From Monastery to Hospital*, 39.

[10] Crislip, *From Monastery to Hospital*, 3.

[11] Crislip, *From Monastery to Hospital*, 8.

[12] Crislip, *From Monastery to Hospital*, 8. Crislip further notes that "the health care system stands among the defining characteristics of Christian monasticism, in evidence from the very beginnings of monastic social organization in the early fourth century. It attracted the notice of contemporary commentators and monastic theorists alike. Its breadth of treatments, its organizational scope, and its guarantee of compassionate care throughout the life cycle set monastic health care in stark contrast with the healing affording in nonmonastic society." Crislip, *From Monastery to Hospital*, 9.

[13] Crislip, *From Monastery to Hospital*, 99.

the ecclesiastical hierarchy in the late fourth century and thus into the preexistent system of ecclesiastical charities"[14]; it was simply a step in the already developing philanthropy of Late Antiquity and the early Middle Ages.

Again, though, the transition to care for outsiders took time. The evolution in the creation of monastic hospitals began in the Coptic monasteries of Egypt, where the traditions of Egyptian and Greek healing continued: "Coptic monasteries thus drew on Egyptian healing traditions that may be traced far into the pre-Christian era."[15] While many similarities can be drawn from the Egyptian and Greek traditions, it was the new monastic infirmary (*infirmarium, pma nnrôme etšône, nosokomeion*) that stood out among the Coptic monasteries, which, "offered inpatient hospital care under the supervision of trained health care providers, including a nursing staff and doctors."[16] The infirmary was probably a complex similar to the Roman military infirmary, but lack of physical evidence does leave us guessing what the earliest infirmaries looked like. We are pretty certain, though, that the infirmary was a separate building and most likely removed from the other buildings for the practice of disease contagion.

By the fifth century CE, writers in both the East and West talk about hospitals, using the term *nosokomeion*, or "place for the care of the sick,"[17] and referring to the infirmaries first created under the Egyptian Coptic monks. Much of what we know about the monastic hospital comes from Pachomius, the founder of Coenobic monasticism, and the *Life of Pachomius* (324 CE), which records that, "after establishing the administrative structure of the monastery, '[Pachomius] appointed another house of stewards to give comfort to all the sick brothers with attentive care according to their rules, and over them a housemaster (*oikiakos*) and a second (*deuteros*) in the same way.'"[18] The infirmary was made up of three major components—all of which dictate the basis for infirmary care throughout the Middle Ages: inpatient facilities,

---

[14] Crislip, *From Monastery to Hospital*, 100.

[15] Crislip, *From Monastery to Hospital*, 32. For more on Coptic Medicine, see Martin Krause, "Papyri Coptic Medical," *CE*, 1886–1888. For more on Ancient Egyptian medicine, see Nunn, *Ancient Egyptian Medicine*.

[16] Crislip, *From Monastery to Hospital*, 10.

[17] Crislip, *From Monastery to Hospital*, 102.

[18] Crislip, *From Monastery to Hospital*, 11.

professional medical care for its patients, and care out of charity.[19] The doctors who provided professional medical care were both male and female, they were highly trained in care, dietary therapy, hygiene, pharmaceuticals (*material medica*), and surgery, and lived along side the monastics in a manner similar to the monks themselves.[20] Nurses, or stewards, aided the doctors. Some monastic infirmaries had an overseer, or elder, who took care of practical administration and who were akin to the masters of the later medieval hospitals.

These first monastic hospitals were monastic and meant first and foremost to care for the brothers. Pachomius himself was on the fence regarding care for the sick outside of the monastic setting. According to his life,

> there was a serious out-break of pestilence in that village, and many people died of it. He would go out to serve them: he would distribute to them a great quantity of wood that he carried from the forest. There was in fact a great and abundant forest of acacias nearby. In short, he served them until God should grant them the favor of healing. When they had been cured of their sickness he said to himself, 'This service of the sick in the villages is no work for a monk. It is only for the clergy and the faithful old men. From this day on, I will no longer undertake it, lest another should put his hand to this task and should be carried away by the scandal of my example, and lest the written word be applied to me, A soul for a soul.' For it is also written, Pure and unspoilt religion in the eyes of God our Father this: to visit the orphans and widows and to keep oneself uncontaminated by the world.[21]

Yet, as monasticism grew, its outlook changed. In all, monastics differed greatly from the governments of the later Roman Empire. As noted earlier, governments and patrons focused on the city, not the people. If healthcare was required, it was done at the homes of those who could afford it. While there were temples to gods, public healthcare was non-existent. Monasticism changed this, regardless of Pachomius' personal beliefs: "In contrast with the medical obsession that had so consumed members of the aristocracy, monastic leaders wrestled less with the

---

[19] Crislip, *From Monastery to Hospital*, 101–102.

[20] Crislip, *From Monastery to Hospital*, 14.

[21] *Pachomian Komonia, Vol. 1: The Life of Saint Pachomius and His Disciples*, trans. Armaund Veilleux (Kalamazoo: Cistercian Publications, 1980), 29.

interpretation of sickness within their own bodies than with the treatment of the sick within society, that is, the healthcare system. Monastic leaders developed systems for providing health care to all monastics and incorporated all manner of sick and disabled individuals into monastic society."[22]

This being said, it should be noted that there was no sudden appearance of healthcare; there was no single person who invented it. Rather, "the monastic health care system was a function of monasticism's unique social organization, its structure and scale, and its isolation from the rest of society. That is, the monastic health care system did not 'develop'; it was a systemic necessity, an unavoidable structural feature of the monastic system"[23] that slowly came about.

For the first true hospital, we look to Basil of Caesarea,[24] and his Basileias or Basiliados.[25] Basil merged the traditions of the monastic hospital and the role of the bishop as father of the poor in his hospital. Basil founded his hospital shortly after he became bishop of Caesarea in 370 CE: "but when I came near enough to Caesarea to observe the situation, refraining, however, from visiting the city itself, I took refuge in the neighboring poor house."[26] The hospital was founded just outside the city; why this being so, however, is unclear, although it was a site of sizeable land. While it seemed to mimic other Christian charities, it differed in its services and architectural complexity,[27] namely it simulated the monastic infirmary.

The Basileias is numbered among the first of hospitals because of its mix of professional care, facilities, and charitable care, all components of the monastic infirmary. Unlike the monastic infirmary, the Basileias provided for outsiders: the poor, strangers and homeless, orphans, the elderly and infirm, lepers, and the sick. As described by Crislip, "many of these social services were traditional Christian activities, undertaken both informally by lay Christians and formally as a function of the episcopal

---

[22] Crislip, *From Monastery to Hospital*, 39.

[23] Crislip, *From Monastery to Hospital*, 41.

[24] Crislip, *From Monastery to Hospital*, 103.

[25] See Sozomen 6.34; Firmus of Caesarea, *Ep. 43* (SC 340). While there is some debate as to if this was indeed the first hospital, it is clear that this is the first hospital for which significant evidence survives. See Crislip, *From Monastery to Hospital*, 103.

[26] *Ep.* 150, tr. Deferrari, alt. in Andrew T. Crislip, *From Monastery to Hospital*, 190.

[27] Crislip, *From Monastery to Hospital*, 104.

office, though some came to the fore only in the fourth century. *All* (*sic*) these services, traditional and novel, were brought together in Basil's hospital."[28]

The Basileias, in its time, was praised for its philanthropy and innovation. Gregory of Nazianzus (d. 389) claimed Basil's hospital to be "a wonder greater than the Colossus that put even the Pyramids to shame."[29] While putting the Colossus to shame is a remarkable feat, "it is in the realm of health care that Basil made his greatest contribution. Indeed, Basil's contemporaries point overwhelmingly to his concern for the sick as the truly distinct aspect of his charity."[30] Basil made it okay to be concerned with disease; he destigmatized it; he made it socially acceptable. Most importantly, he opened his hospital to the general public. As explained by Crislip, "Basil did not invent the hospital, nor did any of his Arian rivals. Nor was the hospital adapted from temples of Asclepius, military or slave valetudinarian, clinics, or public physicians. Rather, the hospital appeared once the monastic health care system was incorporated by Basil, and no doubt by other less celebrated bishops, into the traditional charities of the church."[31] The next big transition would come in the high Middle Ages.

The ideas regarding monasticism, care for the poor, and hospitals eventually made their way to the West where Benedictine Monasticism prevailed. Although later medieval hospitals would adapt the Augustinian Rule,[32] early monasteries who cared for the sick tended to gravitate to the Benedictine Rule (528 CE), which, like the rules of Pachomius, dictated care for the monks primarily. The fourth chapter of the Benedictine Rule lists 'good works', which includes efforts related to the seven works

---

[28] Crislip, *From Monastery to Hospital*, 105–106.

[29] Crislip, *From Monastery to Hospital*, 118.

[30] Ibid.

[31] Crislip, *From Monastery to Hospital*, 140.

[32] It should be noted that while the Benedictine *Rule* was most widely used and followed in early Western Christendom, most hospitals and associations of men and women in hospitals later followed the Augustinian *Rule*. The Augustinian *Rule* does not provide the detail that Benedict's *Rule* does on caring for the sick, but the Augustinian *Rule* emphasizes cleanliness and requests that, when needed, a doctor should be consulted. The Augustinian *Rule* also allows a sick brother to have whatever from the pantry that is seen as necessary for his recovery. See *The Rule of Saint Augustine*, "Chapter Five: The Care of Community Goods and Treatment of the Sick," Robert Russell trans., from Luc Verheijen, *La regle de saint Augustin, Etudes Augustiniennes* (Paris, 1967).

of mercy, such as "14. To relieve the poor. 15. To clothe the naked. 16. To visit the sick. [and] 17. To bury the dead."[33] The good works are adapted from Matthew 25:36 in the Christian Bible: "before and above all things, care must be taken of the sick, that they be served in very truth as Christ is served; because He hath said, "I was sick and you visited Me,"[34] and, "as long as you did it to one of these My least brethren, you did it to Me.""[35] Per the request in Matthew 25:40, the Benedictine Rule responded that the "sick themselves [...] are served for the honor of God, and let them not grieve their brethren who serve them by unnecessary demands. [The demands] must, however, be patiently borne with, because from such as these a more bountiful reward is gained."[36] Finally, Benedict instructed that the "Abbot's greatest concern [...] be that they [the sick] suffer no neglect."[37]

Benedict also addressed how care for the sick was to occur. The sick were to have separate cells and attendants were to serve them.[38] They were to be bathed unless they were young or otherwise healthy; otherwise, bathing was to occur only rarely.[39] The sick were to be offered meat, but as soon as they had returned to health, they were to "abstain from meat in the usual manner."[40] Finally, Benedict warned that the "Abbot exercise the utmost care that the sick are not neglected by the Cellarer or the attendants, because whatever his disciples do amiss falleth back on him."[41] Neglect of the sick reflected poorly on the abbot, and subsequently on the monastery.

---

[33] See also Benedict, *The Holy Rule of St. Benedict*, trans. Reverend Boniface Verheyen (1949), accessed 17 May 2017 at http://www.kansasmonks.org/RuleOfStBenedict.html#ch4. For more on Benedictianism, see Marilyn Dunn, *The Emergence of Monasticism: From the Desert Fathers to the Early Middle Ages* (Oxford: Blackwell Publishing, 2003), 111–137.

[34] Matthew 25:36, NSV.

[35] Matthew 25:40, NSV. See also Benedict, *The Holy Rule of St. Benedict*, trans. Reverend Boniface Verheyen (1949), accessed 17 May 2017 at http://www.kansasmonks.org/RuleOfStBenedict.html#ch36.

[36] Benedict, *The Holy Rule of St. Benedict*.

[37] Ibid.

[38] Ibid.

[39] Ibid.

[40] Ibid.

[41] Ibid.

These rules, however, were aimed at the brothers. Chapter 53 of the Benedictine Rule addresses hospitality to outsiders, proclaiming "Let all guests who arrive be received like Christ for He is going to say, 'I came as a guest, and you received Me' (Matt. 25:35). [...] As soon as a guest is announced, therefore, let the Superior or the brethren meet him with all charitable service."[42] In addition, "in the reception of the poor and pilgrims the greatest care and solicitude should be shown, because it is especially in them that Christ is received."[43] Although the Rule of Benedict tells the brethren to receive and welcome the sick and poor, it does not mention provisions of care, leading one to believe that the concept of the Basileias had not yet reached the West.

Indeed, during the eighth and ninth centuries, monks continued to provide healthcare, to their own. By this point, the monastic hospital had evolved to cater "to three types of the infirm: the superannuated, who slept in the dormitory; the sick, for whom a special room was set apart 'for dangerous illnesses,' meaning perhaps also contagious diseases that could be isolated here; and those who had let blood and shared for a few days the relaxed discipline and richer fare of the infirmary."[44] Eventually, the monastic hospital transformed into a "long building subdivided into four rooms into a large open hall, a dominant form of ward construction under both religious and lay auspices until the eighteenth century,"[45] the design with which most associate modern hospitals. While some parts of the hospital were open to lay members, "the monks' infirmary was closed to lay participants."[46] While this same design would continue into the high Middle Ages, the concept of the Basileias was clearly not embraced in the West under Benedictine Monasticism. Still missing from the equation was the concept of *caritas* and lay participation.

---

[42] Ibid.

[43] Ibid.

[44] Thompson and Goldin, *The Hospital: A Social and Architectural History*, 11.

[45] Thompson and Goldin, *The Hospital: A Social and Architectural History*, 15.

[46] Thompson and Goldin, *The Hospital: A Social and Architectural History*, 11.

## THE IMPORTANCE OF SECULAR CARE: *AMOR CIVICUS* AND *CARITAS* COMBINED

From the chaos of the decline of the Roman Empire emerged many changes, among which was the birth of a gift-giving society. As stated by Patrick J. Geary, "the idea of gift exchange as a fundamental bond of early medieval society is hardly a new concept,"[47] but the increase in lay gifts of land signified a major change in healthcare system practices. Previously, pagan temples, like the temple to Apollo, received treasure but did not need endowed land since the government provided for the temples. In the early Middle Ages, though, with the collapse of a centralized government, those creating centers of care needed concessions, exemptions, and endowments to fund healthcare,[48] especially when not part of the monastic system.

Although monks had been the guardians of healthcare in Late Antiquity, the tradition slowly began to evolve and penetrate into the ranks of secular rulers, as is shown with the lay endowment of a hospital in 542 by King Childebert I, the son of Clovis (d. 511 CE).[49] Childebert I gave funds for the creation of the hospital in Lyons. The hospital, or the Hôtel-Dieu, became the oldest hospital in France, and it was protected under the Fifth Council at Orléans (549 CE). The council threatened excommunication to anyone who embezzled or took the funds that Childebert had provided.

Not long after, other hospitals emerged. The Hôtel-Dieu of Paris, for example, was founded in 651 CE by Bishop Landeric of Paris (d. 661 CE), although he was most likely operating under the charter of Clovis

---

[47] Patrick J. Geary, *Living with the Dead in the Middle Ages* (Ithaca: Cornell University Press, 1994), 77. Regarding earlier works on gift-giving in the early Middle Ages, see Georges Duby, "Taking, Giving and Consecrating," in *The Early Growth of the European Economy*, trans. Howard B. Clarke (Ithaca, NY, 1974), 48–57; Marcel Mauss, *The Gift: Forms and Functions of Exchange in Archaic Societies*, trans. Ian Cunnison (New York, 1967).

[48] The uniqueness of the church, charity, and endowments led to the idea of the municipal hospital within the context of the city. This is key later when we discuss land endowments to the hospital of Saint John. The endowments were a type of piety.

[49] Georges Goyau, "Councils of Orléans," *The Catholic Encyclopedia*, Vol. 11 (New York: Robert Appleton Company, 1911), accessed 8 September 2008 at http://www.newadvent.org/cathen/11318a.htm.

II (d. 657).[50] In a charter of 654, for example, Clovis II confirmed a privilege by the bishop for the monastery of Saint-Denis.[51] He probably did the same for the hospital in Paris, contributing simultaneously to the city and to *caritas*.[52] Although the Hôtel-Dieu preceded the hospital of Saint John in Brussels by over 500 years, its connection to Saint John hospital would be pivotal in its later developments. The Hôtel-Dieu of Paris received its statutes, borrowed from Saint John hospital, in 1220.[53] The statutes would be key in its later municipal developments.

These trends continued over the next few hundred years with one significant change. The fall of the Roman Empire, the rise of the Byzantine Empire, and the cultural, religious, and political split between East and West complicated all matters of life between 500 and 843. The year 843, however, witnessed the "Triumph of Orthodoxy," the end of Byzantine Iconoclasm, and the restoration of icons to the Eastern Church, which subsequently ended one of the great dividing debates between East and West and opened up discussion, trade, and exchange. This was the "revival of regular contacts between emperor, pope and patriarch," which "created a climate in which political and cultural exchange could once again flourish."[54] While transmission of cultural ideas thrived, we can be sure that the Byzantine concept of the hospital made its way to the West.

Byzantium became a key conduit in the transmission of medical practices not only to the Muslims[55] but also to Western Europe.

---

[50]For more on Clovis II's charters, see Barbara H. Rosenwein, *Emotional Communities in the Early Middle Ages* (Ithaca: Cornell University Press, 2006), 146.

[51]The charter, as noted by Rosenwein, uses the terms *timor* and *amor*, going back to the ideas of love for one's city. See Rosenwein, *Emotional Communities*, 146.

[52]The Hôtel-Dieu of Paris remains the oldest hospital in Paris up to this day, as well as the oldest hospital still in operation worldwide.

[53]While 1220 is a fairly firm date, others have suggested that the Hôtel-Dieu may have received the statutes as early as 1217 or as late as 1221. See below for more information.

[54]*Rome Across Time and Space: Cultural Transmission and the Exchange of Ideas, c. 500–1400*, eds. Claudia Bolgia, Roasmond McKitterick, and John Osborne (Cambridge: Cambridge University Press, 2011), 236.

[55]By and large, some of the most sophisticated medical practices and treatises were those of the Greco-Arabic tradition. This includes the work of *Ibn Rushd*, or Averroes (1120–1198 CE), a physician in Moorish Spain, *Al-Razi*, or Rhazes (865–924 CE), a Persian physician, chemist and alchemist and *Hakim Ibn Sina*, or Avicenna. Avicenna wrote The Canon of Medicine. Later, Avicenna's works, as well as those of other scholars, were transmitted into the West through Muslim Spain and via the Crusades. Avicenna's Canon was

More importantly, perhaps, was the fact that the concept of the hospital itself, the *xenones*, similar to the Basileias, made its way to the West from Byzantium. Byzantine hospitals were well ahead of Western ones; "Byzantine hospitals (*xenones*) had begun to focus exclusively on caring for and curing the sick as early as the fourth century A.D.; these philanthropic centers continued to expand their medical services, especially during the reign of emperor Justinian (527–565)."[56] In 843, the "Triumph of Orthodoxy" occurred, which opened up cultural transmission between the West and East, and during which the concept of the *xenones* appeared in the West. It is thus no surprise that "by the eleventh and twelfth centuries they [the Byzantine hospitals] had become the principal theaters of the Byzantine medical profession, providing both specialized treatment to hospital patients and walk-in clinical services to the general population,"[57] while during the same period, an explosion in similar institutions occurred in the West.

The Byzantine hospital was tied closely to the Greek tradition, and the Byzantine hospital, which focused "solely on curing their patients, do not fit the image that twentieth-century historians of medicine and medievalists have presented of premodern hospitals—an image of poorly equipped almshouses more concerned with comforting the sick in their distress than providing medical cures."[58] As Timothy Miller argues, "Christian philanthropy and scientific medicine were indeed wed,"[59] even if it is not at the level that the figures of the Enlightenment would desire it to be.[60]

While much of the traditions in terms of healing practices remained the same, centralized care grew among the Byzantine institutions. One

---

used widely in European medical schools. *National Library of Medicine*, "Islamic Culture and the Medical Arts: Hospitals," accessed 10 August 2016, https://www.nlm.nih.gov/exhibition/islamic_medical/islamic_12.html.

[56] Miller, *The Birth of the Hospital in the Byzantine Empire*, xi. I have chosen to focus on Miller's Introduction to the 1997 edition of his texts as an overview of Byzantine hospitals, as the introduction succinctly presents his arguments in a fashion that is useful for summary. Miller also answers some of the questions raised by the critics of the first edition and posits new questions for ongoing research, both of which are relevant to this work.

[57] Miller, *The Birth of the Hospital in the Byzantine Empire*, xi.

[58] Ibid.

[59] Miller, *The Birth of the Hospital in the Byzantine Empire*, xii.

[60] While Miller presents this argument here for Byzantine hospitals, I will present a similar argument for Western hospitals in the later chapters.

of the pieces of evidence that Miller uses to prove that Byzantine hospitals were indeed medically advanced, and one of the aspects of the Byzantine hospital that goes on to influence the medieval Western hospital, are hospital regulations, or for the lack of a better term, rules. In particular, he talks of one such text, the Pantokrator[61] Typikon (*typika* is a Greek monastic rule[62]) and how it describes "how many physicians and medical assistants were to staff the hospital, how these medical professionals worked in monthly shifts, how much pay they received as compensation for their work, and even how these professional employees advanced to the higher ranks of the medical staff."[63] These are precisely the provisions of care that were missing in the Rule of Saint Benedict.

[61] The most prominent of the Byzantine hospitals was that of the Pantokrator Xenon. Critics of Miller have argued that his work on Byzantine healthcare has relied too much on this particular institution, whereas the other *xenones* might not have exemplified hospital care as the Pantokrator did. Most maintain that the Pantokrator Xenon was unique. Miller combats these ideas with an argument that finds parallels in the West. There exist sources that talk about the Pantokrator Xenon as ideal, but not the exemplar among the hospitals of Byzantium (see, for example, the *vita* of Empress Eirene—*Vita imperatoris Irenes* in Robert Volk, *Gesundheitswesen und Woltätigkeit im Spiegel der byzantinischedn Klostertypika*. Miscellanea Byzantina Monacensia, 28. Munich: Institut für Byzantinisik, neugriechische Philologie, und byzantinische Kunstgeschichte der Universität Müchen, 1983, 191). This is similar to Jacques de Vitry's account of hospitals in the West. Miller also shows that the Pantokrator Xenon was indeed not unique, and there were hospitals that both copied and outdid it. For more on Miller's view of the Pantokrator Xenon, see Miller, *The Birth of the Hospital in the Byzantine Empire*, 12–29.

[62] For more on Greek monastic rules, see Robert Volk, *Gesundheitswesen und Woltätigkeit im Spiegel der byzantinischedn Klostertypika*. Miscellanea Byzantina Monacensia, 28. Munich: Institut für Byzantinisik, neugriechische Philologie, und byzantinische Kunstgeschichte der Universität Müchen, 1983.

[63] Miller, *The Birth of the Hospital in the Byzantine Empire*, xiii. For more on the Pantokrator Typikon, see Paul Gautier, "Le typikon du Christ Sauveur Pantocrator," *REB* 32 (1974), 1–145. The rules are incredibly similar to those of the hospitals of the West during the high Middle Ages, addressing the habits of the brothers, election of the superior, care for sick brothers, occupations within the hospital ward, etc. We do know, for example and in comparison, that the Hotel-Dieu of Paris paid its physicians to treat the patients. We know this from the hospital statutes, and we can assume from this that most places did something similar. Paris had in-house doctors who served the patients: "*donec sanitati restituatur*" while the physicians at the hospital of Saint John could only be called in particular instances. This was probably due to the major difference in size. *Statuta domus Dei Pariensis*, Cap. 21, accessed 17 November 2017, http://rosenwelten.de/stud_hist/editionen/paris.html.

Historians of Byzantium hospitals are more fortunate in showing the clear existence of the medical profession, as the typikon normally detailed such work. Indeed, we know that hospital physicians worked in shifts back to the seventh century CE in Byzantium. We also know that they charged a "high price for private visits. As a result, most people in Constantinople, both the poor and the middle class, came to the hospitals for treatment."[64] Many people also visited the *xenones* to procure medicines.[65] Constantinople even had an officer who supervised all the hospitals of Constantinople.[66]

The state and particularly the emperor in Byzantium founded many *xenones*, distinguishing Byzantium from Rome. Yet, as Miller explains, "we know that private individuals of the fourteenth and fifteenth centuries opened hospitals during the very period in which the emperors were forced to cut back on their support of imperial philanthropic institutions."[67] It would seem that in the West, the Christian lay supporters took up the mantel earlier, i.e., twelfth century, because changes in society necessitated that they care for the poor, whereas in Byzantium, the situation did not compel the involvement of the laity until the fourteenth century. This being said, support for hospitals in Byzantium was supplemented by the "church, the monastic movement, wealthy families, and the medical profession itself."[68]

These advances, however, would have to wait in the West; the newly developing hospitals suffered with the eighth- and ninth-century Viking, Saracen, and Magyar invasions.[69] With the disruptions of the invasions,

[64] Miller, *The Birth of the Hospital in the Byzantine Empire*, xv.

[65] Timothy S. Miller, *The Birth of the Hospital in the Byzantine Empire*, xvi.

[66] Timothy S. Miller, *The Birth of the Hospital in the Byzantine Empire*, xvii. See specifically, the writings of Nicholas of Cusa (1401–1464) who met a Turk who was described as *supermus praeerat hospitalibus*. This suggests that there was even a transference of efforts from the Byzantines to the Muslims. See Miller Timothy S. Miller, *The Birth of the Hospital in the Byzantine Empire*, xvii–xviii.

[67] Timothy S. Miller, *The Birth of the Hospital in the Byzantine Empire*, xvii. This evidence comes to us from Philotheos Kokkinos, the Patriarch of Constantinople from 1354 to 1355.

[68] Timothy S. Miller, *The Birth of the Hospital in the Byzantine Empire*, xviii. There is evidence of wealth patrons and even the poor and sick who later come back to donate to the hospitals.

[69] The *Vita Notgeri episcope Leodiensis* is a poem from the period of the invasions in which the author of the poem assigns the role of the protection of the poor to the bishop. Legislation from the ninth and tenth centuries also insists on the bishop in this role. See Pierre de Spiegeler, *Les Hôpitaux et l'Assistance à Liège (Xe-Xve Siècles): Aspects Institutionnels et Sociaux* (Paris: Sociéte d'Edition "Les Belles Lettres," 1987), 39.

it would take some time before the institutions evolved into what could be consider a "modern hospital." The beginning of that transition can be located in the high Middle Ages and the so-called twelfth-century renaissance. When hospitals reappeared, they would be under the Augustinian Rule, which merged the worlds of the monks and the needy.

## MEDIEVAL MEDICINE

In between the development of the early medieval monastic hospital and the high medieval municipal hospital, significant advances occurred in terms of medical practices. Although the purpose of this book is not necessarily to discuss medical developments, a few key advances should be noted, especially in basic care and obstetrics, as both would be relevant to the developments occurring in Brussels later on. The innovations, however, did not begin in Brussels, but rather in southern Italy, where, from approximately the mid-eleventh century to the thirteenth century, an explosion of medieval activity occurred. Location was key: "southern Italian medicine was characterized by the adoption of practices, theories, and texts coming out of the Arabic world, which added a new patina of science to earlier empirical traditions."[70] It would also be the first to provide medical licenses.[71]

The first writer to make available the advanced Arabic practices was a Benedictine monk, Constantine the African (d. before 1098/99 CE).[72] Constantine translated several medical texts into Latin, including the works of Galen and established a number of works at Montecassino, including, but not limited to, the *Pantegni* (what a physician should know), the *Practica* (who the physician should treat infirmities), the *Book of Degrees* (simple medicines), the *Book of Fevers*, the *Book of Urines*, *On Women's Matters*, Glosses *on Herbs and Spices*, *Surgery*, and *Book of Medicines for the Eyes*. These, and other texts, were studied and disseminated throughout Europe, leading to a revival in medical practices.

The innovative medical practices, however, remained largely removed from the monastic hospital, whose main concern was for the soul. There,

---

[70] *Medieval Italy: Texts in Translation*, eds. Katherine L. Jansen, Joanna Drell, and Frances Andrews (Philadelphia: University of Pennsylvania Press, 2009), 311.

[71] *Medieval Italy: Texts in Translation*, 323.

[72] For more on Constantine, see Peter the Deacon, "Biography of Constantine the African," in *Medieval Italy: Texts in Translation*, 312–314.

patients were given basic treatments, including those most employed by the earliest of peoples; cleaning, bandaging, and plastering/setting bones. Herbal remedies[73] were provided and prayers, or invocations to Christ, were said in a manner similar to ancient temple incubation. Otherwise, actual medical treatment was limited. Some understanding was advanced thanks to dissection, especially of pigs—as dissecting humans as a practice had died out during the Hellenistic period and was not revived until the thirteenth century.[74]

Perhaps the most pertinent advances came in obstetrics. Dissection, surprisingly, filled in some of the unknowns when it came to women's health, organs, and pregnancy. In particular was a better understanding of the uterus:

It is known that nature arranged this organ in women so that whatever superfluity of the whole body is generated in them might be sent through this organ at the accustomed time, just like bilge-water, and hence women naturally have menstruation. This organ is, moreover, the field of our nature, which is cultivated so that it might bear fruit. [For] just as sometimes into good soil there is thrown seed which clings to life [and] which through the action of Nature—with the heat working together and the spirit mediating inside—splits open in the manner of a grain and send out little branches, so certain roots or mouths infix the [human] seed into the uterus and administer nutriment to it and to the fetus being formed.[75]

Furthermore, once the child was born, the "umbilicus" was tied off by the midwife at "the length of four fingers."[76] The fact that the midwife performed this act is key, as a sexual division of labor relegated "aspects

[73] See, for example, the works of Matthew Platearius, *Circa instans*. Matthew was the chief authority on pharmaceutical ingredients, or *material medica*. His work survives in hundreds of extant copies in Latin and many other translated into a variety of European languages. Matthew Platearus, *Circa instans*, in *Medieval Italy: Texts in Translation*, 316–321.

[74] The pig was believed to be "similar in their internal structures, in regard to the position of the internal organs none were found so similar [to humans] as pigs." Matthew Platearus, *Circa instans*, in *Medieval Italy: Texts in Translation*, 321. Most of what was known was through Galen, as identified above.

[75] Copho (attributed), "Anatomy of the Pig," in *Medieval Italy: Texts in Translation*, 322.

[76] Copho (attributed), "Anatomy of the Pig," in *Medieval Italy: Texts in Translation*, 322–323.

of women's medicine to female practitioners out of the concern with morality."[77]

One of the most famous female practitioners was Trota (or Trocta), who composed the compendium, *On the Treatment of Diseases* (c. 1180–1200). Her work, especially on gynecological and obstetrical practices, was hands-on, and demonstrated advanced knowledge, especially in child birthing practices. Included in her work was a section on inducing and hastening birth, which required both herbal and surgical practices. A plant, the marsh mellow—not to be confused with the fluffy white confection today—was boiled. The woman then was to inhale the vapors, while the remains of the plant were placed on her pubis. The treatise suggests inducing sneezing and if necessary, the cutting of the perineum to hasten birth. Trota also provided instruction for purgation after birth and for pain caused by birth.[78]

## CONCLUSION

It is without a doubt that women of the high Middle Ages—midwives, practitioners, and even nuns—followed Trota's advice and saw to the care of all kinds of patients under their watch. The advances of the medieval medicine allowed institutions to provide better services to their patients, even if their expertise was limited by the knowledge of the period. Although profound, the changes that grew out of the early Middle Ages, including but not limited to the rise of the monastic hospital, the transmission of Byzantine ideas, and the rise of medical care, marked a turning point in the creation of municipal hospitals. The Basileias was the example that the West needed to better develop their hospitals. When the hospital did develop in the West in the high Middle Ages, it would transform into the general hospital open to the public, run by government and religious figures, and subsidized by private individuals via charity. It is to those developments that we now turn.

---

[77] *Medieval Italy: Texts in Translation*, 323. Some women did receive medical license, which, as indicated by Jansen, Drell, and Andrews, came through practice.

[78] Trota (?), "Obstetrical Excerpts from the Salernitan Compendium," in *Medieval Italy: Texts in Translation*, 314–315.

# CHAPTER 4

# High Medieval Charitable Institutions and Hospitals, c. 1000–1300 CE

**Abstract** This chapter considers the rise of urban hospitals, their creation, their support, their administration, and their importance. Although still a religious institution, the medieval hospital transformed from a hospice and way station for pilgrims—as had been the case with the early monastery hospital—to a center for care of the urban poor and sick. Care was still overseen mostly by monks and nuns but greater public involvement, especially in administration, emerged. Moreover, the creation of the urban hospital was made possible through lay donations. The Peace of God Movements and the movements to live as Christ's apostles spurred Christians from all levels of society to donate to an urban hospital focused on *caritas* in a manner akin to the Byzantine Basileias.

**Keywords** *vita apostolica activa* · *mater misericordiae* · Urbanization · Regular canons · Municipal hospitals · Donations

## INTRODUCTION

The high Middle Ages has been characterized as the age of hospitals.[1] Increased urbanization, new industrial accidents, famine, and more all provided a presence and a visibility to sickness and the

---

[1] Edward Kealey, "Hospitals and Poor Relief, Western Europe," in *Dictionary of the Middle Ages*, ed. Joseph Strayer (New York: Charles Scribner's Sons, 1989), 6: 293.

© The Author(s) 2018
T. A. Ziegler, *Medieval Healthcare and the Rise of Charitable Institutions*, The New Middle Ages, https://doi.org/10.1007/978-3-030-02056-9_4

poor.[2] As the need for healthcare and charity began to increase, most of the burden of healthcare still fell upon the monasteries.[3] Monasteries by the twelfth century were, however, overtaxed and burdened, and most monastic complexes, even those as large and wealthy as Cluny, could no longer support the load placed on them by the recent developments in society.[4]

Although the Benedictine monks were the primary monastic group in the early medieval West, the transition to the high Middle Ages saw the rise of new reformed monastic orders such as those at Cluny, Cîteaux, and Premontre. The rise in new orders came with the rise of urbanization and many of the new orders fled to the wilderness to escape growing secularization. The newly reformed orders were pivotal, in that they sought to separate themselves from the secular world but continued to provide healthcare. Cistercian abbeys, for example, "have references to hospitals for the laity (*infirmitorium seculare*)."[5] Cluny had an office of the almoner that was in charge of hospice for strangers.[6] These orders, however, could be argued to have practiced a type of charity that was more symbolic than ameliorative, as they were separated from the population that most needed care. This proved problematic given the agricultural revolution, the rise in population, and urbanism. Crowded in the confines of a city, the poor and sick became increasingly visible. For the first time since the fall of the Roman Empire, socially displaced poor and sick people began to plague the streets of European cities. These people were victims of the success of urbanization.[7]

---

[2] In addition, during the eleventh and twelfth centuries, much of Europe experienced widespread famine and disease, which generated greater need among the poor and sick. For example, the *Chronicle* of Sigebert of Gembloux [1126] "mentions 'a great famine in Flanders and many paupers dead of hunger.'" See Mollat, *The Poor in the Middle Ages*, 60.

[3] Pierre de Spiegeler, *Les Hôpitaux et l'Assistance à Liège*, 169–208.

[4] Mollat, *The Poor in the Middle Ages*, 87.

[5] Emily Jamroziak goes on to explain that these were probably located outside of the monastery. She also notes that "such institutions appeared to be a frequent fixture across Europe, but the relationship between 'medical' hospital and hospitals as shelters for the poor is much debated." See Emily Jamroziak, *The Cistercian Order in Medieval Europe: 1090–1500* (New York: Routledge, 2013), ebook.

[6] Gert Melville, *The World of Medieval Monasticism: Its History and Forms of Life* (Collegeville: Cistercian Publications Liturgical Press, 2012), 174.

[7] See especially, Lester K. Little, *Religious Poverty and the Profit Economy in Medieval Europe* (Ithaca: Cornell University Press, 1978).

New urban hospitals arose at a rapid rate, and they owed their creation to various members of the medieval community who made endowments and donations: kings, ecclesiastical lords, burghers, and confraternities who shared in the idea that they were all part of one big "commonwealth."[8] Crucial in this transition was the explosion and involvement of regular canons, many of whom followed the Augustinian Rule, within the urban atmosphere. The Augustinian Rule, similar to the Benedictine Rule, made provisions for the treatment of the sick. While it could be assumed that the rule focused first on the brethren, the location of the canons meant that treatment of the sick extended beyond the walls of a monastery. Regarding charity, the Rule of Augustine states, "charity, as it is written, *is not self-seeking* (1 Cor 13:5) meaning that it places the common good before its own, not its own before the common good. So whenever you show greater concern for the common good than for your own, you may know that you are growing in charity. Thus, let the abiding virtue of charity prevail in all things that minister to the fleeting necessities of life."[9] In regard to care of the sick, the rule specifies, "whether those in convalescence or others suffering from some indisposition, even though free of fever, shall be assigned to a brother who can personally obtain from the pantry whatever he sees is necessary for each one," suggesting care for outsiders.[10] Thus, the rise of the canons and the involvement of the laity meant that the hospital movement was not necessarily a full-fledged lay movement, as many of those who sought to aid the sick and poor did so under religious vows. Indeed, the religious element never left; rather the focus changed.

The real origins of the medieval hospital lie in community spirit and a desire to help one's neighbor. In their aspirations to help create hospitals, many members of the lay community returned to the Church Fathers and the Gospels, initiating the movement most often titled the *vita apostolic activa*.[11] If you could not or were not able to live as 'Christ's poor', then your next best choice was to provide for the poor and sick. Moreover, the new focus on the Virgin Mary made the transition complete—love for the neighbor rather than love for God became

---

[8] Kealey, "Hospitals and Poor Relief, Western European," 6: 293.

[9] Augustinian Rule, chapter 5.

[10] Ibid.

[11] André Vauchez, *The Spirituality of the Medieval West from the Eighth to the Twelfth Century*, trans. Colette Friedlander (Kalamazoo: Cistercian Publications, 1993), 86.

paramount. The movement toward medieval communalization flourished with the introduction of hospitals. The most affluent of society founded hospitals; other Christians simply provided donations in varying amounts.

In this process of providing to burgeoning institutions of healthcare, there was little distinction between a charitable donation and a business transaction, and thus little distinction between public and private. Whereas someone or a group may certainly have benefited financially or otherwise from a donation, lease, or rent, the nature of the transaction was nearly always spiritually motivated, and there was often a counter gift, either in the form of continued prayer, or in more tangible benefits to the donor: "the way of access to sanctity was [...] the practice of charity."[12] Stephen White argues that "by giving alms, men could supposedly attain salvation after their deaths. Almsgiving entailed an exchange process in which humans gave away the transitory earthly wealth [...] in return for an eternal inheritance in God's kingdom."[13] This exchange happened through intermediaries, such as monks and the lay hospital staff who became the "clients of the saint to whom the community was dedicated and whose network of patronage radiated outward."[14]

The simple equation that giving and providing influenced salvation created a new-found success for charity and healthcare in the form of the urban hospital.[15] By the twelfth century, the monopoly that the church and monasticism had once held on healthcare had been broken: "laymen were no longer content to rely on clerics and monks to perform works of charity on their behalf."[16] Instead, poor care became more and more communal and centralized, which forced healthcare and charity away from the authority of the institutionalized church and into the hands of municipal authorities.[17]

---

[12] André Vauchez, *The Spirituality of the Medieval West from the Eighth to the Twelfth Century*, 130.

[13] Stephen D. White, *Custom, Kinship, and Gifts to Saints: The Laudatio Parentum in Western France, 1050–1150* (Chapel Hill: The University of North Carolina Press, 1988), 155.

[14] White, *Custom, Kinship, and Gifts to Saints*, 29.

[15] Kealey, *Medieval Medicus*, 83.

[16] Mollat, *The Poor in the Middle Ages*, 95.

[17] For an alternative view, see R. I. Moore, who argues that "where money reigned supreme, the growing and increasingly menacing presence of the poor pointed to the necessity of providing for their control and, if necessary, their confinement or expulsion

## THE URBAN HOSPITAL

Prior to the high Middle Ages, the monastery was the locus of care, while the regulation of the monastic hospital had been under the auspices of the abbey and abbot. The advent of the high Middle Ages, however, witnessed the rise of other types of hospital-like institutions, including, but not limited to, leper houses, almshouses, and hospices for travelers and pilgrims,[18] the regulation of which varied. Most towns also had guild almshouses and private almshouses, as well as separate hospitals for Jews, the insane, and for lay "gentlefolk,"[19] such as the "infirm and aged."[20] Although healthcare varied according to the institution, the majority of people cared for at the emerging 'hospitals' were people who had a "need" in society, but not a particular medical aliment,[21] similar to those seeking care in Late Antiquity. This included "pilgrims, the blind, [the disabled], elderly priests or impoverished, children, and honest tradesmen who had fallen on hard times."[22] It was from this institution of care that the ancestor of the modern hospital, the urban municipal hospital, was born.

from the community." R. I. Moore, *The Formation of a Persecuting Society* (Massachusetts: Blackwell, 1990), 106. Thus, it should not come as a surprise that many hospitals, especially leprosarium, were located outside the city walls. The hospital of Saint John, however, was an exception to this rule.

[18] *The Hospital in History*, Granshaw and Porter, 21.

[19] Clay, *The Medieval Hospitals of England*, 23. The so-called gentlefolk could move around as they pleased from ward to private room, where as those with plague or disease were limited to the confines of their ward. Money could buy privacy, and the elderly with means could use hospitals as a kind of retirement home.

[20] de Spiegeler, *Les Hôpitaux et l'Assistance à Liège*, 112.

[21] Carole Rawcliffe, *Medicine and Society in Later Medieval England* (Phoenix Mill: Alan Sutton Publishing, 1995), 205.

[22] Rawcliffe, *Medicine and Society in Later Medieval England*, 205. Edward Kealey further notes that hospitals "could be centers for poor relief; clinics; dispensaries; homes for indigent students; hostels for travelers; leprosaria for people of all ages and classes; residences for the blind, the elderly, the mentally ill, and the orphaned; and the multi-department complexes with large professional staffs." See Edward Kealey, "Hospitals and Poor Relief, Western Europe," in *Dictionary of the Middle Ages*, ed. Joseph Strayer (New York: Charles Scribner's Sons, 1989), 6: 294.

Urban hospitals, at least at first, were scarce; the care of the sick was often seen as an "unwelcome or impossible burden,"[23] the latter being the greater deterrent. Once created, though, like other institutions connected to the Christian faith, most urban hospitals received structural and financial backing from the church. Because of their urban character and because the church and municipal councils were inextricably linked, most municipal hospitals also received monetary assistance from the city council. Typically, urban hospitals were under the control of the bishop,[24] but they were also "semi-independent institution[s], subject to royal and episcopal control in matters of constitution, jurisdiction and finance, yet less trammeled in organization than most religious houses."[25] At times, these hospitals would be tied to the parochial system; almost always, though, the institution had a connection to monastic life, be it through care or regulation[26]; this is no surprise, given the history and the transmission of ideas regarding healthcare and institutions, especially from the Byzantine Basileias.

Similar to their early medieval predecessors, high medieval hospitals for the sick were normally provided with statutes and regulations. Most often, the statutes included a *regula*—to be discussed below.[27] The conferral of a rule required proper religious authority, which was done typically by the diocesan bishop.[28] This is not to say, though, that the bishop had complete control over the institution. Although the bishop could be seen as an administrator of religious matters, it was secular authority that granted rights of temporal privilege, such as immunity from taxation.[29] The secular authority could be a king, an emperor, a local duke, or even the town alderman or city council.

---

[23] *The Hospital in History*, Granshaw and Porter, 25.

[24] A range of hospitals existed in terms of authority. Some hospitals did not have a permanent altar or were not dependent on Episcopal authority. See de Spiegeler, *Les Hôpitaux et l'Assistance à Liège*, 106.

[25] Clay, *The Medieval Hospitals of England*, 211.

[26] Ibid.

[27] See above for more on the Benedictine Rule, used in early medieval monastic hospitals, and the Augustinian Rule, used in later hospitals.

[28] Clay, *The Medieval Hospitals of England*, 194.

[29] Clay, *The Medieval Hospitals of England*, 194–195. Furthermore, "royal interest helped multiply the numbers of doctors, hospitals, and medical books, and this expansion gave health care a higher governmental priority than it might otherwise have enjoyed." Kealey, *Medieval Medicus*, 25.

Most hospital units remained small.[30] The average hospital might have a dozen beds, whereas larger hospitals could care for as many as 200 people.[31] Regardless of size, the usual hospital consisted of rectangular wards that characterized the open-ward system, which was adapted from the similar monastic design.[32] Often, the ward was attached to other buildings, such as a church or cathedral. This too was a holdover from the previous monastery hospital.[33] One major change to the open-ward system was a *T* or *L* layout, which allowed inmates to view the altar, the host, and communion from their bed. The *L* or *T* layout also allowed the people who provided care to the sick to live separately from the sick. Halls then radiated from the infirmary, providing access to the living quarters. Some hospitals began with small open wards and grew bigger over time by adding more wards or cross wards. Saint John's hospital in Bruges (c. 1188), for example, was a small open-ward hospital that increased in size by adding more and more wards.[34] The plan was ideal and oriented to the growing population; if overcrowding occurred, which it frequently did, the patrons could easily add cross wards.[35]

[30] James Brodman explains that one can get a sense of size from inventories. See Brodman, *Charity and Religion*, 62.

[31] *The Hospital in History*, Granshaw and Porter, 26. Although the most prevalent, the open-ward style was not the only one. Greek and Roman wards designed around an open courtyard did exist as discussed earlier. Many hospitals did indeed take this form, but even so, the open-ward system was by far the preferred choice. See Kealey, *Medieval Medicus*, 84.

[32] The open-ward system was "taken over from the monasteries, adapted, enlarged, refined, and eventually mass-produced. [...] The form prevailed for nearly four centuries." Thompson and Goldin, *The Hospital: A Social and Architectural History*, 20–21.

[33] The location of most of the early modern hospitals was next to or near a cathedral cloister, but in later periods, hospitals began to appear elsewhere. Because of the possibility of disease and contamination, some hospitals were built in undesirable areas, and typically the institutions were located outside city walls in order to contain disease. In other cases, especially in those of the leprosaria, the institutions were located along the rivers and waterways. Brodman, *Charity and Welfare*, 62. For more on leprosaria and the reaction of the public, see R. I. Moore, *The Formation of a Persecuting Society*, 42–56. Finally, to insure security, safety, and order, many hospitals were surrounded with a wall and a towered gate.

[34] Thompson and Goldin, *The Hospital: A Social and Architectural History*, 24.

[35] Such was the case of the hospital de Santa Cruz in Barcelona in the fifteenth century, which had four large halls that all opened into one another and into a large hall. See Thompson and Goldin, *The Hospital: A Social and Architectural History*, 30.

In addition to the ward, most hospitals had a chapel, and commonly had one or more altars. Similar to altars in other religious houses, hospital altars had oil lamps with rush wicks and wax tapers burned before them all day. The altars proved necessary, as daily life simply could not be separated from religious life in a hospital.[36] Indeed, secular and religious life often merged: "from warden to pauper, all were expected to pay strict attention to the faith and give themselves to devotion[;] all who could rise attended the chapel on bended knees, the bedridden worshipping simultaneously. Even the sick people could join in the intercessions."[37] Despite the assimilation from secular to religious life, hospital inmates were still distinguished from hospitals workers and were clothed in a uniform of "coarse warm clothing [that] was readily distinguished from the ragged mendicant."[38] In addition, patients typically slept on straw pallets, while "wooden bedsteads were probably introduced late in the twelfth century."[39] Other amenities included bedding and hanging lamps.[40]

Central to the hospital was the chapel, which provided a constant visual reminder of *caritas* and the hospital founders and benefactors.[41] Before a hospital could construct a chapel, the institution and its administrators received special permission from the bishop certifying that it did not interfere with the parochial system.[42] The need for episcopal approval rarely deterred hospital staff from building a chapel, since the chapel was an important source of income. Many donors made contributions on the condition that masses would be celebrated for them.[43] The funds received from the chapel were then used for oblations, while agreements were made regarding public worship on certain occasions in

---

[36] Clay, *The Medieval Hospitals of England*, 158. Hospitals were often adorned with religious paintings and carvings in the chapels, often of patron saints and many had religious books and religious implements, such as plates and vestments. It should not come as a surprise that "many valuables fell a (*sic.*) prey to dishonest wardens." Clay, *The Medieval Hospitals of England*, 164.

[37] Clay, *The Medieval Hospitals of England*, 158.

[38] Clay, *The Medieval Hospitals of England*, 176.

[39] Clay, *The Medieval Hospitals of England*, 172.

[40] *The Hospital in History*, Granshaw and Porter, 29.

[41] de Spiegeler, *Les Hôpitaux et l'Assistance à Liège*, 193.

[42] Clay, *The Medieval Hospitals of England*, 197.

[43] de Spiegeler, *Les Hôpitaux et l'Assistance à Liège*, 193–194.

the chapel.[44] Without the chapel, many hospitals would have ceased to function for lack of funds, and without a chapel, the hospital's Christian mission may have been diminished.

In addition to the brothers and sisters, hospitals were run by lay volunteers and appointed staff. Volunteer workers who served the hospital received no salary, but did receive food and clothing.[45] In exchange for food and clothing, the volunteers worked in the hospital doing various tasks. Women typically saw to the bedside needs of the patient, in addition to other "domestic duties,"[46] such as cleaning and laundry. This means, then, "actual care of the sick poor in hospitals was the responsibility of the sisters or women servants."[47] Male volunteers and brothers tended to religious and administrative duties, such as prayers and donations.

Both brothers and sisters of the hospital followed the *Rule* of Saint Augustine,[48] as noted above, while most of the volunteers, the sisters, and the brothers wore Augustinian robes, which were black or brown, had a cloak and hood, and a cross on the outside. Jacques de Vitry (1160/70–1240 CE), a contemporary in the high medieval hospital movement, served as both a witness to and critique of the rise of the medieval and early modern hospital. Jacques argued that ideal hospitals should be organized based on the *Rule* of Saint Augustine, not that of Benedict. He insisted that hospitals be placed under church control and be modeled on the example of the Hospitallers.[49] Thus, the move from monastery to town did not remove the religious element of the hospital, but it did change it. No longer was the focus on the Benedictine Rule; now the hospital looked to the more open Augustinian Rule.

Initially, the Middle Ages supported two types of hospitals: monastic hospitals where the regulation is under the control of the abbey and hospitals under the control of the bishop; in these two categories are a range of hospitals, many of which did not have a permanent altar or who were not dependent on Episcopal authority.[50] The monastic hospitals were the

---

[44] Clay, *The Medieval Hospitals of England*, 197.

[45] Clay, *The Medieval Hospitals of England*, 152.

[46] See Clay, *The Medieval Hospitals of England*, 154.

[47] *The Hospital in History*, Granshaw and Porter, 32.

[48] See Kealey, *Medieval Medicus*, 108–109.

[49] de Spiegeler, *Les Hôpitaux et l'Assistance à Liège*, 112.

[50] de Spiegeler, *Les Hôpitaux et l'Assistance à Liège*, 106.

main caregivers in the early Middle Ages, but they were later replaced by municipal institutions supported by members of both the monastic and lay community. When we do get to the civic hospitals, they varied in composition and power.[51] The new hospitals of the twelfth century (leprosarium and confraternal hospitals) appear as a break from both early medieval monastic hospitals and ancient hospitals. At this point, there was a greater adoption of the Augustinian Rule to control the hospitals; was certainly the case in Liège.[52] Some hospitals, however, moved beyond the Rule of Augustine, as it provided spiritual directives, but not organizational ones; thus, it had to be "adapted and developed."[53]

Although the Rule of Saint Augustine was meant for monastic communities, it was open to some interpretation.[54] The rule provided spiritual directives, but not organizational ones; thus, it had to be adapted. Most of the time, the rule was amended into the hospital's statutes. The statutes of the hospital determined the roles of the people involved in care and also the daily religious observances, food and clothing allowances, and types of conduct.[55] If the rules were not followed, penalties such as flogging, fasting, fines, stocks, suspension, and expulsion could be applied.[56]

While the brothers and sisters worked in hospitals, they did not always run them; this was a major change that seems to follow the traditions of the Greek East and Byzantium. At the head of the institutions were various officials whose power varied according to the institution's mission. These leaders included, but were not limited to, priests, *mambours*,[57] almsmen, and wardens, who were akin to the monastic abbot, and masters, and mistresses. The warden, usually, but not always, a priest,[58] often

---

[51] De Spiegeler notes that the power of the city in association with the hospital varied from city to city. de Spiegeler, *Les Hôpitaux et l'Assistance à Liège*, 122.

[52] de Spiegeler, *Les Hôpitaux et l'Assistance à Liège*, 147.

[53] Ibid.

[54] de Spiegeler, *Les Hôpitaux et l'Assistance à Liège*, 135.

[55] Kealey, "Hospitals and Poor Relief, Western Europe," 6: 295.

[56] Clay, *The Medieval Hospitals of England*, 138.

[57] de Spiegeler, *Les Hôpitaux et l'Assistance à Liège*, 133.

[58] Clay, *The Medieval Hospitals of England*, 149. In the case of Saint John's hospital in Brussels, the masters and mistresses were brothers and sisters of the hospital community.

also served as the master of the hospital.[59] Masters did not offer phys-ical cure; they offered spiritual care. Masters, similar to early Christian bishops, were obliged to visit the poor twice per week and the sick twice per day. During the visits, the master was not allowed to be squeamish, regardless of malady; instead, he was to be merciful and benign.[60] In addition, the master had little time for leisurely activities: "he conducted certain services both in the chapel and parish church, and kept school, besides ruling the alms house,"[61] which kept him present not only dur-ing the day but at night as well.

Masters were "the most visible members of hospital staff,"[62] whereas "physicians were neither mentioned as members of hospital staffs, nor did they figure prominently in early hospital statutes."[63] If medical treat-ment was provided, it was done by either a physician[64] (*phisicus, fisicus*), surgeon (*cirurgicus*), apothecary (*apothecaries, speciarius, herbolarius*), barber (*barberius, barbitonsor*), or healer (*medicus, metge* (in Catalonian documents)).[65] Most physicians[66] were only brought in on an as needed

---

[59] The warden/master was drawn from the ranks of the brothers, and was also known as "prior, *custos*, keeper or rector." Norman Moore, *The History of St. Bartholomew's Hospital*, Vols. I and II (London: C. Arthur Pearson Limited, 1918), 288.

[60] Clay, *The Medieval Hospitals of England*, 150.

[61] Clay, *The Medieval Hospitals of England*, 151. Although a much later example, a fifteenth-century founder regulation displays some of these characteristics. It instructs that the master of Ewelme "must be an able and well-disposed person in body and soul, one who could counsel and exhort the poor men to their comfort and salvation. He had to conduct frequent services, and was warned to omit none—not even 'for plesaunce of lorde or lady.'" Clay, *The Medieval Hospitals of England*, 151. In another example, we learn of a basic function of the master as the person responsible for overseeing the acquiring and pur-chasing cloths for the hospital: "William Hardel, Mayor of London in 1215–16, was witness of a charter of Alexander of Norfolk, in which he grants to St. Bartholomew's Hospital, his house outside the gate of St. Paul's, toward the sought and opposite the brewery of the cannons of St. Paul's in the parish of St. Gregory. With its rent they are to buy the clothes necessary '*in tulchia magna hospitalis*' for the poor staying there at night—according to the direction of the master." Moore, *The History of St. Bartholomew's Hospital*, 320–321.

[62] Kealey, *Medieval Medicus*, 104.

[63] Kealey, *Medieval Medicus*, 105.

[64] Edward Kealey provides a table of the known physicians in England from 500 to 1154. See Kealey, *Medieval Medicus*, 31.

[65] Brodman, *Charity and Religion*, 86.

[66] James Brodman explains that "by the thirteenth century, there [were] signs that med-ical care was being introduced into a few institutions. [...] The Hospitaller Order of Saint John [was] particularly influential in this development because, as early as its statues of

basis,[67] most hospitals simply worked to keep patients alive, and most patients did not typically undergo aggressive treatment.[68]

Treatments included bed rest, cleaning of wounds, setting of bones, and a good diet.[69] Some patients were bled and some were purged; otherwise invasive treatment meant the setting of fractures, binding, and suturing wounds, dressing sores and rashes, and fixing dislocations, similar to early medical care. Although the aforementioned treatments could be performed by a male or female, women were the major care givers, especially when it came to obstetrics and gynecology.[70] This made the role of the female particularly important in the hospital.

Typically, the hospital master was aided by other officials, as well as a "proctor," who was the financial agent of the community and the bearer of the official seal.[71] The seal was "to be kept under three keys, of which one [was] to be kept by the master of the hospital and the other two by two brethren nominated by the master and brethren on the advice of the prior, but the prior [was] not to have power to remove these key keepers."[72] The proctor was assisted by a collector, who, when collecting alms, had to swear only in the name of the hospital; all money received was then rendered to the hospital brothers. Finally, most hospitals also

1182, the order maintained four physicians at its large hospital in Jerusalem to diagnose disease and prescribe medicine." Care such as this only arrived in Catalonia, Spain, by the end of the fourteenth century. Even so, "records of late medieval hospitals show that the sick comprised substantial proportions of the inmate population, indicating that the transformation of these institutions from mere shelters to facilities dispensing medical care was indeed well underway." See Brodman, *Charity and Religion*, 93.

[67] The Augustinian Rule argued that "if the cause of a brother's bodily pain is not apparent, you make take the word of God's servant when he indicates what is giving him pain. But if it remains uncertain whether the remedy he likes is good for him, a doctor should be consulted." *The Rule of Saint Augustine.*

[68] Brodman, *Charity and Religion*, 96.

[69] *The Hospital in History*, Granshaw and Porter, 31. Rarely did the leper or almshouses provide medical care. Also, the institutions specifically designed for travelers and pilgrims typically did not provide care. *The Hospital in History*, Granshaw and Porter, 24.

[70] Rawcliffe, *Medicine and Society in Later Medieval England*, 194.

[71] Sometimes it was left to him to deliver a sermon, so his role was both spiritual and administrative. When the traffic in indulgences began, the proctor became a "pardoner." Clay, *The Medieval Hospitals of England*, 153.

[72] Moore, *The History of St. Bartholomew's Hospital*, 378.

had what were called "under-officials," clerks in minor orders who might assist in worship and work.[73]

In addition to the master and the proctor, hospitals had a rector, or a *procurer* who was chosen by the bishop or municipal council because he was a respectable member of the community. The procurer oversaw the administration of the hospital and had to maintain discipline and order by controlling illicit behaviors of the various hospital administrators.[74] The *procurer* had the ability "to withhold salaries, to impose fines, and to inflict corporeal punishment."[75] If the *procurer* was in an order, he maintained priestly duties as well.[76] Some *procurers* served for life, while others were only appointed for fixed terms.

## CONCLUSION[77]

The most important change in the evolution from monastery hospital to municipal hospital was in the care of the inmates themselves and in the administration of the institution. Religion remained a key component

---

[73] Clay, *The Medieval Hospitals of England*, 155.

[74] Brodman, *Charity and Religion*, 50.

[75] Brodman, *Charity and Religion*, 51. There were times, however, obedience fell to the job of the warden: "On the next day but one after Hugh's death the king committed to Brother Maurice, chaplain of the house of the Temple in London, the care and keeping of the Hospital of St. Bartholomew till the king with his justiciar should come to London and arrange more fully as to the ruling of the same, and the brethren and sisters of the hospital were commanded meantime to be attentive and obedient to the aforesaid Brother Maurice as to their warden." Moore, *The History of St. Bartholomew's Hospital*, 373.

[76] Brodman, *Charity and Religion*, 51. With so many duties, it should not come as a surprise that some hospitals were prosperous and others were not. Brodman, *Charity and Religion*, 53.

[77] James Broadman wrote in his 2009 book, *Charity and Religion in Medieval Europe* that "the High Middle Ages gave birth to the ancestor of the modern hospital." He goes on to note that "the term *hospital* is to be understood by its root meaning—that is, as a place of shelter rather than a locus of care—every town and many villages and rural locales came to possess one or more of this institutions." Finally, Brodman argues that most hospitals were tied to their local communities and that the "initiative for their foundation can be attributed to no single segment of medieval society, for we can count among their benefactors, bishops cathedral chapters, monasteries and religious orders, and pious laypeople, as well as religious, professional, and municipal associations." Brodman, *Charity and Religion in Medieval Europe*, 45. Concerning these observations—ancestors to modern hospital, places of shelter, and multiple initiatives in founding—Brodman cannot be

of the hospital care, but exactly who received care and how changed. Prior to the twelfth century, monks, rather than municipal authorities, were prominent in hospital care, primarily of their own members. Later, though, charity became linked to urban centers and their authorities. No longer was care of the sick and poor a concern of only monks. Now, aldermen, rectors, priests, and wardens joined into care for the less fortunate. This transition was possible as *caritas* through the *vita apostolica activa* moment became connected to local trustees.[78] Thus, as transition occurred, public hospitals became connected to city centers and gained more prominence in urban landscapes. The municipal hospital still relied largely on regular canons, Augustinian brothers and sisters, and others for care, but increased lay involvement via donations made a significant contribution to the numbers and success of the high medieval hospital.

Urban hospitals relied principally on private aid in the form of gifts or donations from private patrons. Some gifts were in kind; others were in specie. Most of the donations came from annual rents raised on lands and property that were then provided to the hospital. Many hospitals also had endowments in kind, such as grants from royal forests,[79] and even rights to the water dripping from the gutter between the houses.[80] Hospitals also received money from bequests, participated in trade, and held fairs. They collected admission fees from people who were newly admitted members of the institutions, from the alms of pilgrims, and from involuntary funds, such as a Hospital Sunday Fund, or tolls on produce or other items. Voluntary donations came largely from fraternities who oversaw the maintenance of the charities.[81] The increase in lay

disputed. Although participation in the management of the hospitals could be achieved by a multitude of peoples, including secular governments, it is Brodman's belief that episcopal governments ran the hospitals: "secular municipal institutions were too immature before 1200 or 1300 to challenge, supplant, or augment episcopal initiatives. Thus, it was almost by default that the bishop had to become the father of the poor." While in some cases the role of the bishop was paramount, in others, it was not. The hospital of Saint John was certainly one such exception, and it is through it and the others that mimicked Saint John that the true municipal hospital was born. See Brodman, *Charity and Religion*, 46–47.

[78] Clay, *The Medieval Hospitals of England*, 17.

[79] See de Spiegeler, *Les Hôpitaux et l'Assistance à Liège*, 181; Moore, *The History of St. Bartholomew's Hospital*, 339.

[80] Moore, *The History of St. Bartholomew's Hospital*, 401–402.

[81] Clay, *The Medieval Hospitals of England*, 183–191.

concern for the poor and ill prompted patrons from nearly every level in society to donate. The result was an affluence of hospitals in the high Middle Ages and the creation of the urban hospital most akin to today's institution.

The public municipal hospital had made its debut. As an institution, it was unique to the urban centers of the high Middle Ages, yet still connected to its monastic brother of the past. While many would argue that the later hospitals of the Reformation became the basis for modern institutions, it was the high medieval urban hospital that deserves the title. The traditional monastic hospital after which the high medieval hospital was designed was supposed to be dedicated to the care of the poor and to the care of those who could not provide for themselves; yet, by the fourteenth century, "the tendency to differentiate among classes of the poor is evident [...]. There were those whose condition, age, or status required services beyond mere asylum; some hospitals were reserved for specific classes of individuals, like aged fishermen, impoverished priests, or abandoned children."[82] Later, more specialized hospitals began to emerge, and societies began to create hospitals that were reserved for certain groups of people, i.e. "good children" or poor patricians.[83] The trifold make-up of the traditional hospital—professional care, inmate facilities, and charity—had disappeared.

The true urban hospital of the high Middles did not discern, thereby making it a more fitting ancestor of today's modern hospital. The medieval hospital did not exist without a chapel and it did not exist without its benefactors, both of which were seeped in notions of *caritas*. The hospital of Saint John in Brussels exemplified inclusion in terms of both treatment and benefactors. It is to the specific case of the Hospital of Saint John in Brussels that we turn to understand this very development.

---

[82] Brodman, *Charity and Welfare*, 64.
[83] Mollat, *The Poor in the Middle Ages*, 152.

# PART II

# Case Study of the Hospital of Saint John

# CHAPTER 5

# The Creation of the Hospital of Saint John

**Abstract** Although the early hospital movement had created a number of hospitals, many of the institutions remained rural in character. Other monastic hospitals were overtaxed and overburdened. The creation of the Saint John's signaled a new hospital that merged the urban charitable institutions and the monastic hospital into one coherent unit, especially through its statutes. The statutes were clear, concise, and orderly, but they also guaranteed the bishop's power. This resulted in a local church–state debate. Occurring simultaneously throughout Europe was a greater church–state debate that sought to reform religious institutions, including hospitals. Saint John's statutes were used, borrowed, and disseminated among the episcopal networks in the local and immediate area, making it a standard example of the municipal hospitals of the high Middle Ages.

**Keywords** Hospital of Saint John · Brussels · Bishop of Cambrai · Statutes · Duke of Brabant · Castellan

While Saint John hospital would go on to influence many nearby and neighboring institutions, its influence was rather limited due to the confines of geography. Most influence would be in the northern regions of Europe, particularly in the areas of modern-day France, Brussels, and Germany. Other hospitals in Italy, Southern France, Spain, the Holy Roman Empire, and beyond emerged without the influence of Saint John hospital in Brussels, and became important in their own right.

© The Author(s) 2018
T. A. Ziegler, *Medieval Healthcare and the Rise
of Charitable Institutions*, The New Middle Ages,
https://doi.org/10.1007/978-3-030-02056-9_5

## INTRODUCTION

Early in its history, Brussels followed the pattern of most medieval cities by providing charitable establishments that cared for the poor and pilgrims: the institutions of Saints Julien, Carmel, Jacques, and Laurent all saw to the basic needs of travelers and the less fortunate such as sustenance, shelter, and basic care. The hospital movement, however, did not arrive in Brussels in full force until the twelfth century. In Brussels, the hospital of Notre-Dame-et-des-douze-Apôtres—later named the hospital of Saint-Gertrude—appeared sometime before 1127 and was located near the church of Saints-Michel-et-Gudule.[1] Two years after the foundation of the hospital of Notre-Dame-et-des-douze-Apôtres, the hospital of Saint Nicholas emerged near the Grand' Place, the central square of Brussels where major public offices and markets could be found. Sometime before 1162, the hospital of Saint Jacques arose near Coudenberg Palace, the home to the Dukes of Brabant, while the leprosarium of Saint Pierre appeared in 1174. Finally, in 1186, the confraternity of Saint-Esprit, the confraternity from which Saint John's hospital was formed, came into existence.[2]

---

[1] This hospital did not last; later it evolved into a convent. See Paul F. State, *Historical Dictionary of Brussels* (New York: Rowman and Littlefield, 2015), 145.

[2] Aside from brief mentions of Saint John by other historians working on other related topics but not this hospital per se, and by contemporaries commenting on the hospital in travel journals and local studies on the town of Brussels, the hospital of Saint John has only been studied in some detail by two scholars. Both of the studies were done in French, and Paul Bonenfant and his student, Paul Evrard, conducted them. Bonenfant's contribution includes a reconstructed cartulary of the known documents related to Saint John's hospital, several articles, and other related works on poor relief and healthcare. The second important work on the hospital is that of Paul Evrard: an unfinished Master's Thesis. In the introduction to the work, Evrard confirms that a group of priests, clerics, and *bourgeois* (sic.) of Brussels created the hospital. He then explains that the majority in the group of the bourgeois *hardly* responded to the needs for which the group was founded, those same needs that initially drove people to create hospitals based on the seven works of mercy. He argues instead that the members of the groups related to the hospital sought out political and landed aggrandizement. His main focus, however, is on the fourteenth century. See *Cartulaire de l'Hôpital Saint-Jean de Bruxelles* (*Actes des XII^e et XIII^e Siècles*), ed. Paul Bonenfant (Brussels: Palais des Académies, 1953) and Paul Evrard, "Formation, Organization Generale et etat du domaine rural de l'hôpital Saint Jean au Moyen-Age," Unpublished Master's Thesis, Universite Libre de Bruxelles, 1965.

Despite the many hospitals that preceded it, Saint John[3] hospital grew to become the most important hospital in Brussels.[4] It was the only hospital in Brussels up until the *Ancien Regime* to serve as more than just an almshouse, while Saint John hospital and Saint Pierre leprosarium were the only institutions fully open to the public. Saint John hospital served the public indiscriminately, while care at Saint Pierre leprosarium was limited to those afflicted with leprosy.

Despite its profound importance, the original hospital met its demise toward the end of the seventeenth century. In 1695, Marshal of Villeroi leveled the original hospital during a bombardment,[5] but it was rebuilt. Other incarnations of the institution followed in 1843 and in 1950. Today's Brugmann hospital has taken Saint John's place.[6] Although the hospital is no longer standing, the three streets it once occupied still bear witness to its former existence. Located in the area are a pharmacy and other related medical stores. The street names also point to the former existence of the hospital, including "Saint John's Street" and "Hospital Street."

The hospital of Saint John found its beginnings in the twelfth and thirteenth centuries; it owed, however, its existence to the people, events, and structures that had preceded it. The political development of the duchy of Brabant, the religious structure of the diocese of Cambrai, and the social developments of the lay religious movement all informed the birth and development of the hospital of Saint John. The hospital grew to become arguably the most important hospital to the people of

---

[3] Although the hospital is no longer standing, the three streets it once occupied still bear witness to its former existence. Located in the area are a pharmacy and other related medical stores. The street names also point to the former existence of the hospital, including "Saint John's Street" and "Hospital Street."

[4] See de Spiegeler, *Les Hôpitaux et l'Assistance à Liège*, 81.

[5] This bombardment occurred in August 1695 by an army of the marshal of Villeroi. On 11 August 1695, the marshal and his 70,000 forces occupied the area of Anderlecht. As State explains, "the bombardment began on the evening of 13 August. More than 3,000 assorted cannonballs and shot rained down on the city, setting fire to close to 4,000 buildings." While he goes on to note that most of the damages were "made good within five years," the extent of the destruction to archives and some buildings is still being felt. Indeed, it was during this time that the Hospital of Saint-Jean's was destroyed. See State, *Historical Dictionary of Brussels*, 38.

[6] Brugmann hospital was constructed in another location before Saint John's was destroyed. The new hospital was built in 1923 according to the designs of Victor Horta.

Brussels. Its influence, however, stretched beyond the city streets and walls, making it an excellent example of the medieval municipal hospital. Exactly how Saint John hospital achieved these accolades follows.

## HISTORY OF BRUSSELS AND SAINT JOHN HOSPITAL

Urban life did not exist in the Brabant region—which included Brussels—until the tenth century,[7] and when it did come into its own, the medieval town of Brussels found itself to be unlike many of the towns in Northern Europe. Brussels, originating from the word, 'broek-sele',[8] was not able to claim Roman origins,[9] making it a second-generation city.[10] Unable to fall back on Roman beginnings and expand outward, like the cities of Cologne or even Paris, Brussels was forced to develop from the outside in: the agricultural and economic framework came before the city and slowly contributed to its growth.[11] Historians—including Adriaan Verhulst—have argued that the slow pace of urbanization can be attributed to the lack of a large river, which

[7] Adriaan Verhulst explains that there were "no perceptible signs of urban life [in Brabant] until the tenth century." Adriaan Verhulst, *The Rise of Cities in North-West Europe* (Cambridge: Cambridge University Press, 1999), 110. The hospital was first mentioned in the hagiographic source *Miracula sancti veroni*. The source was written between 1015 and 1020 and it called Brussels a "*portus.*" See also Paulo Charruadas, "Croissance Rurale et Action Seigneuriale aux origins de Bruxelles (Haut Moyen Âge-XIIIe siècle)," in *Studies in European Urban History 10 (1100–1800)* "Voisinages, Coexistences, Appropriations: Groupes sociaux et territories urbains (Moyen Âge-16e siècle)," sous la direction de Chloé Deligne et Claire Billen (Turnhout: Brepolis, 2007), 176.

[8] Meaning dwelling on the marsh, settlement on the swamp, and other variations. Bram Vannieuwenhuyze, Paulo Charruadas, Yannick Devos and Luc Vrydaghs, "The Medieval Territory of Brussels: A Dynamic Landscape of Urbanization," in *Landscape Archaeology Between Art and Science*, ed. S. J. Kluiving, E. B. Guttmann-Bond (2012), 230.

[9] For more discussion on this issue, see Edith Mary Wightman, *Gallia Belgica* (Berkeley: University of California Press, 1985); Adriaan Verhulst, *The Rise of Cities in North-West Europe*; and Helen Clarke and Björn Ambrosiani, *Towns in the Viking Age* (New York: Saint Martin's Press, 1991).

[10] Paulo Charruadas, *The Cradle of the City: The Environmental Imprint of Brussels and Its Hinterland in the High Middle Ages* (Springer-Verlag, 2011), 256. See also, *Brussels*, ed. Claire Billen and Jean-Marie Duvosquel (Mercator Fonds: Antwerp, 2000). Most importantly, see Mina Martens, *Histoire de Bruxelles* (Brussels: Privat, 1976). Finally, see Paul Bonenfant, "L'origine des villes brabançonnes et la <<route>> de Bruges à Cologne," *Revue belge de philology et d'histoire* Tome 31 fasc. 2–3 (1953): 399.

[11] Paulo Charruadas, *The Cradle of the City*, 255.

placed Brussels behind other Roman cities. The Romans, for example, traded along the Rhine in Cologne in the first century CE and along the Seine in Paris as early as the third century BCE. Urbanization for Brussels, however, began rather late, around 1000 CE, with the creation of a *portus* on the River Senne.[12] The *portus* established Brussels as an important place of trade since goods had to be off loaded at the port and then carried to and from the city.

Commercial and political growth followed[13] the creation of the *portus* and development was further fueled by the rise of an east–west route from Cologne to Bruges that included Brussels in its path.[14] Brussels had experienced quasi-autonomy in its early history, which was one of the benefits of being a second-generation city. The town and its rural hinterlands encountered little involvement from ecclesiastic[15] and monastic[16] powers as Christianity spread into Northern Europe.

Slowly, the Counts of Brabant, who were also the Counts of Louvain, assumed rulership. The Counts originally designated Louvain as their

[12] Verhulst, *The Rise of Cities in North-West Europe*, 111. See Paul Bonenfant who surveys the birth of the town—from its importance as a port town and town along the route to Cologne to the creation of the *castrum* and commercial development. Paul Bonenfant, "Une capital au berceau: Bruxelles" *Annales. Économies, Sociétés, Civilisations 4ᵉ année*, No. 3 (1949), 298–310. Also, Vannieuwenhuyze, Charruadas, Devos and Vrydaghs "The Medieval Territory of Brussels: A Dynamic Landscape of Urbanization," 226. See also Alexander Henne and Alphonse Wauters, *Historie de la Ville de Bruxelles* (Brussels: Perichon: 1845, 1968); G. des Marez, "Le développement territorial de Bruxelles ua Moyen age," *Congrés International de Géographie Historique*, Tome III, 1935; Martens, *Histoire de Bruxelles*, 1976

[13] Vannieuwenhuyze explains that "unlike, for instance, Flemish cities (Tits-Dieuaide, 1975), Brussels did not require massive imports of wheat before the end of the Middle Ages. Between 1100 and 1300, Brussels became a center for the countryside. At that time, the city functioned as the main market attracting rural production surplus (Charruadas 2007a). This is fundamental in understanding the scope of agricultural expansion in the Brussels area." Vannieuwenhuyze, Charruadas, Devos and Vrydaghs, "The Medieval Territory of Brussels: A Dynamic Landscape of Urbanization," 232.

[14] Bonenfant, "L'origine des villes brabançonnes et la <<route>> de Bruges à Cologne," 400, 447. Ernest Gilliat-Smith, *Story of Brussels* (London: J.M. Dent and Co., 1906), 33.

[15] The nearest centers were in Tournai, Liège, and Cologne. Charruadas, *The Cradle of the City: The Environmental Imprint of Brussels and Its Hinterland in the High Middle Ages*, 257.

[16] Charruadas also discusses absence of bishops and abbots (monasteries and archbishoprics). Due to their absences, this was a period where many of the religious structures were financed by the laity. This will be of particular note later. Charruadas, "Croissance Rurale et Action Seigneuriale aux origines de Bruxelles," 183.

capital, but eventually moved the capital to Brussels.[17] There, the new Counts, considered outsiders, had to purchase lands around the city in order to guarantee the town's growth and economic success.[18] In the process of purchasing lands, the Counts began to make claims to the city's important religious and political foundations, and as a result "were able to put their mark on the religious and administrative infrastructure of the cities."[19] The creation of monastic and canonical networks by the twelfth and thirteenth centuries followed the success brought by the new Counts,[20] while the arrival of monastic and canonical networks[21] in turn contributed to the growth of the region. As the burgeoning city and the rural hinterlands increased, lords and rural elites moved into the town[22]; they formed the rich "bourgeois" or burgher class.[23]

[17] André de Vries, *Brussels: A Cultural and Literary History* (Oxford: Signal Books, 2003), 10. De Vries explains that before the move, the Dukes of Brabant, in order to look after their duchy, appointed "a *bailli* (bailiff), a *châtelain* (castle warden), and an *amman* (administrator)." André de Vries, *Brussels: A Cultural and Literary History* (Oxford: Signal Books, 2003), 28. See also Mina Martens, "Du site rural au site semi-urbain" dans, *Histoire de Bruxelles* (Toulouse, Privat, 1976), 52–55.

[18] Charruadas, *The Cradle of the City*," 259.

[19] Peter Stabel, "The Market Place and Civic Identity in Late Medieval Flanders," *Shaping Urban Identity in Late Medieval Europe*, ed. Marc Boone and Peter Stabel (Leuven: Apeldoorn, 2000), 60.

[20] Paulo Charruadas, for example, has identified the following networks: Affligem within the important parish of Asse, Anderlecht, Brussels, Forest, Grand-Bigard, La Cambre at Ixelles, Jette, Grimbergen, Niewenrode and Petit-Bigard at Leeuw. Charruadas, *The Cradle of the City: The Environmental Imprint of Brussels and Its Hinterland in the High Middle Ages*, 259.

[21] Brussels fell into the jurisdiction of the bishopric of Cambria: "in Brabant, attempts were made in the thirteen, and again in the fourteenth century to separate Brabant from Cambrai and Limburg from Liège. Henry I (c. 1230), Jean II, and especially Jean III (1332 and 1336) urged this, in vain, with the pope." Ludo J. R. Milis, *Religion, Culture, and Mentalities in the Medieval Low Countries: Selected Essays*, ed. Jeroen Deploige, Martine De Reu, Walter Simons, and Steven Vanderputten (Belgium: Brepols, 2005), 83 n1.

[22] The twelfth century was characterized by seigniorial expansion, especially in the second half of the century. The Dukes especially played a huge role in the establishment of these places, as did the rural lords. It is to them that we have to credit the initial foundation/growth of the city. Charruadas, "Croissance Rurale et Action Seigneuriale aux origines de Bruxelles (Haut Moyen Âge-XIIIe siècle)," 187–200.

[23] Charruadas, *The Cradle of the City: The Environmental Imprint of Brussels and Its Hinterland in the High Middle Ages*, 260. "Though the patricians as a body were a wealthy class, all of them were not rich men according to Gilliat-Smith. See Gilliat Smith, *The Story of Brussels*, 41. The qualifier of 'rich' is quite necessary as we now know that

The growth of the town after these developments was great and rapid. By 1138, the Counts of Brabant began appointing magistrates (*échevins*) who were charged to enforce commercial laws.[24] These men were most certainly drawn from the ranks of the burgher class. In 1183, Frederick Barbarossa I (1123–1190 CE) established Brabant as duchy within the Holy Roman Empire. To the Counts of Brabant, he gave the hereditary title of Duke. The Dukes of Brabant were thus indebted to the Empire.[25] Henry I (1165–1235 CE), son of Godfrey III of Louvain (1142–1190 CE), became the first Duke. With their official status, the Dukes of Brabant continued to focus on their capital and granted in 1229 a charter (*keure*) to the city of Brussels and its inhabitants.[26] The charter guaranteed the freedom of the wealthy in the town, and therefore favored the burgher class. Shortly later, in 1235, the Duke of Brabant appointed seven magistrates[27] and thirteen jurors,[28] which again drew from the burgher classes.

As Brussels grew, so too did its wall. The *première enceinte*—two and a half miles (four kilometers) around with some forty towers and seven gates—was created sometime before 1134 and after the construction of Ducal Palace of Coudenberg.[29] While the exact date is uncertain, we do know that by end of the twelfth century Brussels was enclosed by a wall.[30] Estimates suggest that the wall took around eight years to finish[31] and included St. Géry, the Cathedral of St. Gudule, the original

---

"from the thirteenth century onwards, much of the land around Brussels (perhaps over half) belonged to rich city dwellers." See Charruadas, *The Cradle of the City: The Environmental Imprint of Brussels and Its Hinterland in the High Middle Ages*, 259. See also Vannieuwenhuyze, Charruadas, Devos, and Vrydaghs, "The Medieval Territory of Brussels: A Dynamic Landscape of Urbanization," 233. The authors discuss the emergence of urban elite in Brussels.

[24] de Vries, *Brussels: A Cultural and Literary History*, 29.

[25] This proves important later on when the hospital of Saint John becomes embroiled in the fight between the papacy and the empire.

[26] Martens, *Histoire de Bruxelles*, 66–69.

[27] For more on the magistrates, see Martens, *Histoire de Bruxelles*, 58.

[28] The role of the Châtelain declined in the early and mid thirteenth century and was replaced by the aldermen. Martens, *Histoire de Bruxelles*, 63.

[29] Paul Bonenfant, "Les premiers remparts de Bruxelles," *Annales de la Société royale d'archéologie de Bruxelles* (XL, 1936), 46.

[30] Bonenfant, "Les premiers remparts de Bruxelles," 28.

[31] de Vries, *Brussels: A Cultural and Literary History*, 21.

Coudenberg, and the Steenpoort[32] within its confines of its eighty hectares.[33] Six churches, numerous hospitals, and many merchant enterprises existed within the original walls.[34] Later, the hospital of Saint John would make its appearance inside the walls.

Brussels also developed the new quarters of Ruysbroec and Sablon near the outer wall,[35] prompting, for example, the town council,[36] to create a second city wall in the thirteenth century "whose perimeter fixed the urban territory *strictu sensu*."[37] The first gate was mentioned in 1238.[38] Notre-Dame de la Chappell and Saint Catherine Church, two parish churches, were both outside the outer wall.[39] Inside the walls was the city center,[40] including the Grand' Place, the Ducal Palace, the major markets, the town cathedral, and Saint John Hospital.[41] As already

---

[32] de Vries, *Brussels: A Cultural and Literary History*, 14. Also, Georges Despy, "La genese d'une ville," in Jean Stengers et al., *Bruxelles: Croissance d'une capital* (Anvers: Fonds Mercator, 1979), 28.

[33] Despy, "La genese d'une ville," 28.

[34] Ibid.

[35] Claire Dickstein-Bernard, "Activité économique et développement urbain à Bruxelles (XIIIe–XVe siècles)," *Cahiers Bruxellois* 24 (1979): 56.

[36] Appointed by the duke.

[37] The wall remained "until the beginning of the nineteenth century, when it was demolished (Lelarge 2001)." Vannieuwenhuyze, Charruadas, Devos, and Vrydaghs, "The medieval territory of Brussels: A dynamic landscape of urbanization," 232.

[38] Georges Despy, "Un dossier mystérieux: les origines de Bruxelles," *Bulletin de la Classe des Lettres et des Science Morales et Politiques*, 6ᵉ série, Tome VIII (Académie Royale de Belgique, 1997), 286.

[39] Charruadas, "Croissance Rurale et Action Seigneuriale aux origines de Bruxelles (Haut Moyen Âge-XIIIᵉ siècle)," 177. See this page for a plan of the locations of the new inhabitants of Brussels beginning before 1200.

[40] Charruadas, "Croissance Rurale et Action Seigneuriale aux origines de Bruxelles (Haut Moyen Âge-XIIIᵉ siècle)," 180.

[41] Vannieuwenhuyze, Charruadas, Devos, and Vrydaghs, "The Medieval Territory of Brussels: A Dynamic Landscape of Urbanization," 224. Location within or outside the walls dictated the prosperity of the area. The center of prosperity was around the parish of Saint-Nicolas by the end of the fifteenth century. There, only about nine percent of the poor households could be numbered; around Coudenberg, it was eight percent. The area of Notre-Dame de la Chapelle and Saint-Gery saw higher percentages: fifteen percent and fourteen percent, likely influenced by the habitation of textile workers nearby. The greatest poverty was around the chapel of Saint Catherine (twenty-one percent)—most likely this is because the area was periodically ravaged by the flooding of the Senne and by various epidemics. Dickstein-Bernard, "Activité économique et développement urbain à Bruxelles (XIIIe-XVe siècles)," 62.

noted, the hospital of Saint John was not the only nor the oldest hospital in Brussels[42]; several institutions preceded it. These early care centers *were* sufficient for the town's inhabitants during the twelfth century. As, however, the city expanded, Brussels needed an institution dedicated solely to the sick and poor. Saint John hospital, thanks to the timing of the lay movements, would assume that role.

## The Rise of a Municipal Hospital

The Peace of God movements initially and the *vita aposolica activa* and *mater misericordiae* movements later on saw to the care of the poor and the sick[43] and spread throughout Europe to affect the lay population to action. In several Belgian towns, laymen took the initiative to organize charitable enterprises. The city of Brussels was no exception. In 1162, Godfrey III (1142–1190)—Count of Brussels and Duke of Lower-Lorraine—appealed to the Hospitallers in Cologne at Saint James Hospital, beseeching them to establish a similar institution in Brussels. Nothing, however, came of the first appeal. Godfrey III renewed his appeal once again in 1183 when he went on pilgrimage to Jerusalem. In the Holy Land, Godfrey III visited the hospital of Saint John,[44] which

[42] Before 1127, the Hospital of Notre-Dame and of the Twelve Apostles existed. It was first under the patronage of Saint Gudule and later under the patronage of Saint Gertrude. In 1129, a hospital dedicated to Saint Nicholas appeared, while a third hospital, under the protection of Saint James, existed by 1162. Finally, a leprosarium was created sometime before 1174. See Rawlins Cherryhomes, "Charity in Brussels: The Hospital Saint John (1186–1300)" (Unpublished Masters, University of Texas, 1963), 71. "Several hospitals were founded at Brussels before the time of Jacques de Vitry: Notre Dame, entitled Saint Gertrude in the modern period, before 1127; Saint Nicholas, 1129; Saint James, 1162; the leprosarium of Saint Peter, before 1174; Saint John, 1176. Notre Dame and Saint John were staffed by communities of both sexes." John Frederick Hinnebush, *The Historia Occidentalis of Jacques de Vitry: A Critical Edition* (Fribourg: The University Press, 1972), fn 150.

[43] In the early Middle Ages, people took care of sick based on interpretations of James 5:14–15 and the anointing of the sick.

[44] The Hospital of Saint John in the Holy Land was created by the Order of the Knights of Saint John, or the Knights Hospitaller. In the struggles between the Christians and the Muslims in the Holy Land, a hospital was created to care for the sick and injured but to also provide charity for the poor and hospitality to Frankish pilgrims. The hospital was located in Jerusalem, the brothers followed the Benedictine Rule, and the institution was overseen by the Master. As pilgrims migrated to the Holy Land, many joined the institution. The growth of the institution allowed them autonomy as their own institution, and

certainly had been influenced by similar Byzantine and Muslim institutions. This visit inspired Godfrey to create a similar house in Brussels that would be dedicated to the sick and infirm and not just the poor: "*inenarrabilia Spiritus Sancti carismata, que in paupers et imbecilles et infirmos habundanter et humiliter sum erogata.*"[45]

While nothing materialized from Godfrey's efforts in the Holy Land, seeds for a municipal care center in Brussels had been planted.[46] Between Godfrey's attempts and the rising charity movements, it was only a matter of time before Brussels saw the birth of a municipal hospital. The new initiative, however, came not from the nobility but rather from the rising burgher class. The hospital of Saint John's first incarnation was as the confraternity of Saint-Esprit,[47] which was formed by a group of clerics, priests, and burghers: *presbyteris, clericis, burgensibus Bruxellensibus.*[48] The confraternity received official approval from the bishop of Cambrai, Roger de Wavrin (r. 1178–1191 CE), in 1186.[49] The Order of the Hospitallers of the Holy Spirit and the associated confraternity took on characteristics that separated them from their monastic predecessors. Among their concerns was the care of not only travelers and the poor, but also the sick, orphans, abandoned infants, pregnant women, and pilgrims.[50] These new concerns would be central to the developments

under Master Gerard, they established their own order that operated under papal control (*Omne Datum Optimum*, Pope Innocent II, 1139), at which point they took the name Knights Hospitaller. See Steven Runciman, *A History of the Crusades Volume II* (Cambridge University Press, 1952), 156.

[45] Cherryhomes, "Charity in Brussels: The Hospital Saint John (1186–1300)," 73–74.

[46] Godfrey III married Margaret of Limburg (1135–1172) in 1155. Their son, Adalbert, was born in 1166 and went on to become a bishop of Liège.

[47] Paul Bonenfant, *D'Histoire des Hôpitaux* (Brussels: Annales de la Société Belge, 1965), 19. Confraternities in this period were common and stood as "a corporation of members combined in efforts for the increase of social and religious opportunity." *Church and City 1000–1500: Essays in Honour of Christopher Brooke*, ed. David Abulafia, Michael Franklin, and Miri Rubin (Cambridge: Cambridge University Press, 1992), 5.

[48] *Cartulaire de l'Hôpital Saint-Jean*, SJ 2, p. 7. The original is lost.

[49] Bonenfant, *D'Histoire des Hôpitaux*, 19–20. See also Dickstein-Bernard, "Activité économique et développement urbain à Bruxelles (XIIIe–XVe siècles)," 56.

[50] R. P. CH. De Smedt, "L'ordre hospitalier du Saint-Esprit," *Revue des questiones historiques*, Vol. 54 (1 July 1893): 217.

of Saint John hospital.[51] Moreover, nearly all confraternities practiced charity in various forms. The confraternities of the Holy Spirit, however, were particularly devoted to *urban* charity and therefore were often managed by local urban administration.[52] It is thus no surprise to find the request for the confraternity in Brussels to include the 'burgher' citizens, rather than the local monks.

Although the transition is muddy from confraternity to hospital, it is clear that the local authorities, in the case of the dukes, members of the town's administrations, and near-by religious powers, played a role in the subsequent creation of the hospital of Saint John, already giving it a sense of 'municipal' concern. Sometime between 1186 and 1204, Thierry II, the abbot of Jette, and his convent sent members of their community to help with the confraternity,[53] suggesting that the monks

---

[51] *Cartulaire de l'Hôpital Saint-Jean de Bruxelles*, ed. Bonenfant, 5. Cherryhomes informs us that "the origins of the Cologne charity are quite obscure but its existence was mentioned as early as 1175." Cherryhomes, "Charity in Brussels: The Hospital Saint John (1186–1300)," 72. See also M. Reymond, "Les Confreries du Saint Esprit au pays de Vaud," *Zeitschrift fur Schweizerische Kirchengeschichte*, XX (1926), 282–301. The earliest mention of the *fraternitas Sancti Spiritus* in Cologne is 1175; see F. F. Schaefer, *Das hospital zum hl. Geist auf den Domhofe zu Köln* (Köln: 1910). This connection makes sense because of the established trade routes that Brussels had with Cologne. See above.

[52] Michel Mollet, *The Poor in the Middle Ages*, 275. Mollet's discussion of poor tables can be found in his chapter titled "From charity to policing the poor." Although one might think of policing in a negative way, it is not much different from the controlling of the deserving poor that occurred in the Reformation. For more information on "village-confraternity-communities of the Holy Spirit," see Pierre Duparc, "Confraternities of the Holy Spirit and Village Communities in the Middle Ages," *Lordship and Community in Medieval Europe: Selected Readings*, ed. and trans. Fredric L. Cheyette (Huntington: Robert E. Krieger Publishing Company, 1975), 341. The Confraternity of the Holy Spirit in Brussels may have been related to Gui de Montpellier's religious order of the Holy Spirit, but more likely it was simply another local charity that arose due to need in the early thirteenth century. Paul Brune, for example, notes that the confraternity in Brussels was related to the poor tables and not the later hospitals. See Paul Brune, *Histoire de l'ordre Hospitalier du Saint-Esprit* (Paris: C. Martin, 1892), 196.

[53] The document reads as follows: "*Omnibus sancta matris Ecclesie filiis in Christo dilectis, T., Dei patientia Jettensis ecclesie dictum abbas, totusque conventus, salute. Omnem que auctore Spiritu Sancto in Christo fieri solet fraternitatem ac societatem approbari atque laudari dignum esse fatemur, quinimmo illam que in ejusdem Sancti veremur. Nos itaque fraternitatem speciali Sancti Spiritus titulo insignitam Bruxelle cum alacritate et gaudio spirituali suscipimus, omnesque qui in ea ad pauperum ac debilium recreationem elemosinarum suarum amminicula transmiserint, in nostre, fraternitatis societate connumeramus omniumque beneficiorum nostrorum, orationum, missarum, vigiliarum atque elemosinarum participes constituimus.*" *Cartulaire de l'Hôpital Saint-Jean*, SJ 3, p. 8. CPAS SJ 4.

were more than willing to relinquish their role as hospital leaders to others. In the records, Abbot Thierry II names the confraternity as that of the Holy Spirit; the monks of Jette from the order had the implicit goal to help the sick and poor.[54]

By 1195, the confraternity must have made a transition to an institutional hospital; that year the first Duke of Brabant,[55] Duke Henry (r. 1183/1190–1235),[56] in order to encourage bequests and donors, drew up an exemption from military obligations for those who would retire to the hospital. Retirees would be liable for their payments on their fiefs and could no longer engage in their secular trades or pursuits, while the poor table/confraternity-soon-to-be-hospital would inherit their estates. The charter was approved, witnessed, and recognized by a collection of urban authorities, including clerics, a later priest, and the town castellan.[57]

The Duke's exemption found success.[58] In only a few years between Henry's exemption and 1204, the would-be hospital would become an official institution. When exactly this change occurred is not clear. In the 1204 record of military exemption, the word *fraternitatem* had been replaced with *hospitalis*, while the hospital was identified as the organization previously dedicated to the Holy Spirit: "[...] in *hospitali, quod in honore Sancti Spiritus apud Bruxellam edificatum est* [...]."[59]

Because Saint John hospital was in the jurisdiction (*ressort*) of Brussels, it was the responsibility of the duke of Brabant.[60] Henry's

---

[54] *Cartulaire de l'Hôpital Saint-Jean*, SJ 3, p. 8. CPAS, SJ 4, fol. 11.

[55] H. De Bruyn. "Origine de l'Église et de l'hôpital de Saint-Jean, au Marais, a Bruxelles," in *Analectes Pour Servir à l'histoire ecclésiastique de la Belgique*, t. 4 (Brussels, 1867), 31. In addition, an 1846 inscription to be placed on the hospital reads, "*a la pieuse et perpétuelle mémoire de Henri I, duc de Brabant, au fondateur et au plus grand bienfaiteure de l'Hôpital Saint-Jean.*" See *Administration Générale des Hospices et Secours de la ville de Bruxelles*. Hôpital Saint-Jean, 7.

[56] Although dated, the best source for Duke Henry is G. Smets, *Henri I Duc de Brabant 1190–1235* (Bruxelles: Lamertine, 1908).

[57] *Cartulaire de l'Hôpital Saint-Jean*, SJ 4, pp. 9–10. The original is lost.

[58] Gifts, including money donations and patrimonies, given to hospitals were considered "insurance policies that would eventually pay dividends." Kealey, *Medieval Medicus*, 89.

[59] See *Cartulaire de l'Hôpital Saint-Jean*, SJ 4, pp. 9–10. The original is lost.

[60] Mina Martens, *L'Administration du Domaine Ducal en Brabant au Moyen-Âge (1250–1406)* (Brussels: Académie Royale de Belgique, 1952), 416.

commitment to the hospital was apparent[61]: "*Ego, Henricus, Dei gratia dux Lotharingie [...] ad opus pauperum hospitalis beati Johannis, quod antea Sancti Spiritus dicebatur.*"[62] In addition to the above-discussed military exemption, Henry awarded to the poor of the hospital of Saint John the feudal tax (*tonlieu*) that he collected on wood in Brussels. It is clear from the record that the new hospital of Saint John that Duke Henry named was the old confraternity of the Holy Spirit: "[...] *ad [me] pertinent in Bruxella, ad opus pauperum hospitalis beati Johannis, quod antea Sancti Spiritus dicebatur.*"[63] What remains unclear is the reason for the change in saintly patronage, although several factors most likely contributed to the renaming.

Between 1197 and 1198, Duke Henry I undertook a crusade to the Holy Land. He went to Acre and visited the hospital of Saint John, which had been moved from its original location in Jerusalem. Perhaps Henry I, like Godfrey III, was impressed with the hospital in the East, thereby prompting him to rename the pseudo hospital when he returned.[64] Possibly, it was to fall in line with the other nearby confraternity in Cologne that the original confraternity of the Holy Spirit mimicked. The Cologne confraternity's seal, for example, was composed of a scene of Saint John baptizing Christ in the River Jordan[65]; the hospital

---

[61] "*Ego, Henricus, Dei gratia dux Lotharingie [...] ad opus pauperum hospitalis beati Johannis, quod antea Sancti Spiritus dicebatur.*" CPAS, SJ 4, fol. 1.

[62] *Cartulaire de l'Hôpital Saint-Jean*, SJ 5, p. 12. CPAS, SJ 4.

[63] Ibid.

[64] The change in name was not so simple; "it is likely that Duke Henry I, after his crusade to the Holy Land in 1197–1198, imposed the new name without changing the organization of the hospital itself." Henry I, perhaps in imitation of Godfrey, made his way to Acre. After the fall of Jerusalem, Acre became the principal site of the hospital of the Order. They remained in Acre until its fall in 1291. Henry I may have adopted the name thanks to his experience visiting Acre. Finally, the renaming might have been linked to the Brotherhood of Cologne, the confraternity upon which Saint John was imitated. The brotherhood's seal is of Saint John baptizing Christ in the River Jordan. The hospital of Saint John adopted the same seal. See Cherryhomes, "Charity in Brussels: The Hospital Saint John (1186–1300)," 108, 75. Regardless of the origin of the name and patron, Saint John stuck, thereby branding this important institution and its space well into the modern era. Even today, the site of the former hospital is named the Place Saint-Jean.

[65] Bonenfant, *D'Histoire des Hôpitaux*, 20. Bonenfant explains that when the group of Saint-Esprit changed its name to Saint Jean, it was probably (*san doute*) in the imitation of Saint John of Jerusalem.

of Saint John adopted a similar scene for their seal. Conceivably, though, it was just a matter of consolidated ease: Saint John was the patron saint of the adjacent church and thus served as a fitting patron for the new hospital. Regardless, by 1207, the group was completely in the hands of the *fraters hospitalis Bruxellensis* and Saint John was their saint.[66] Following the change, the group beseeched and received protection from the papacy the same year.[67]

In 1207, Pope Innocent III (d. 1216) extended his protection over the hospital brothers and their holdings, as it was not uncommon for monasteries, churches, and religious associations to ask the papacy for protection and for the papacy to grant it. In some cases, however, papal protection was used to overshadow local authority. Godfrey, the then-castellan of Brussels, his wife, Helewige, and his son, Lionnet, the castellan-to-be, had exempted the hospital from annual census payments in January 1209, for example.[68] Similarly, in December 1210, Godfrey honored the erection of a chapel by the parish of Notre-Dame de la Chapelle, which was located not far from the growing hospital in Saint John. The parish of Notre-Dame de la Chapelle must have felt the pressure of the growing hospital, as Godfrey also forbade the hospital to bury in its enclosure.[69] In the meantime, the priest of Forest, Gautier, granted the hospital of Saint John perpetual use of a court located next to the hospital in June 1210,[70] signifying continued aggrandizement by the hospital. Later that month, the Abbot of Afflighem, Robert (r. 1203–1227 CE), approved the priest's transfer.[71]

Saint John hospital would continue to increase in size after the initial foundation. Although the exact size of the hospital remains elusive,[72]

---

[66] Bonenfant, *D'Histoire des Hôpitaux*, 20.

[67] Although normal and not altogether uncommon, papal protection is significant in this case. It is a clear indicator of significant development, as with each new extension of protection, the papacy was protecting more and more of Saint John's holdings.

[68] See *Cartulaire de l'Hôpital Saint-Jean*, SJ 7, pp. 14–16. The original is lost.

[69] Bonenfant, *D'Histoire des Hôpitaux*, 67.

[70] *Cartulaire de l'Hôpital Saint-Jean*, SJ 8, pp. 16–17. CPAS SJ 31.

[71] *Cartulaire de l'Hôpital Saint-Jean*, SJ 9, pp. 17–18. CPAS SJ 31.

[72] There is a serious lack of sources regarding the size of the hospital, the care provided, and the inmates. Much of what can be determined about medieval Saint John hospital has to be distilled from later sources. For more on the sources that do exist, see Tiffany A. Ziegler, "'I Was Sick and You Visited Me:' The Hospital of Saint John in Brussels and Its Patrons" (Unpublished PhD dissertation, University of Missouri-Columbia, 2010), chapter 2, especially 53–60.

a contemporary of Saint John hospital, the hospital of Louvain, had twenty beds by the end of the thirteenth century.[73] Saint John's statutes did allow a doctor to be brought in in cases of *particularis infirmitas*,[74] while during the Burgundian regime (1430–1477 CE), the city surgeon visited the hospital of Saint John once per day and the city doctor once per week.[75] By 1501, an ordinance stipulated that "patients had to be placed in a bed with clean sheets and a blanket and be suitably clothed in the winter."[76] In 1780, Saint John hospital had 135 beds, but it lacked an operating room.[77] By no means was the hospital huge, but it was the newly designated general hospital open to all those who had need in the community.

## Conclusion

Saint John hospital grew rapidly, and as a result, Saint John and other institutions, such as Notre-Dame de la Chapelle, were at odds over territory, parishioner's rights, and jurisdiction. Although the castellan had made some efforts to resolve the disagreements, the dispute eventually garnered the attention of the local bishop. The bishop of Cambrai, John of Bethune (r. 1200–1219 CE), stepped in to formally proclaim his power over the religious institution in 1211, thereby asserting his power over the town's castellan. This was more than a simple debate between church and state regarding a rather small hospital. At the heart of the dispute was the greater struggle between empire and papacy, which pitted the Duke of Brabant, who owed his position to the Holy Roman Emperors, and his castellan against the Bishops of Cambrai, who tended to side with the papacy. At the conclusion of the struggle, the hospital of Saint John would emerge not only as the municipal hospital of Brussels, but also a model for hospitals in the region.

---

[73] John Walter Marx, *The Development of Charity in Medieval Louvain* (New York: Yonkers, 1936), 31. Saint John hospital received its first cemetery in 1237, while the hospital of Louvain did not receive a cemetery until 1260.

[74] Bonenfant, *D'Histoire des Hôpitaux*, 27–28.

[75] State, *Historical Dictionary of Brussels*, 145.

[76] Ibid.

[77] Ibid.

# CHAPTER 6

# On Bishops, Popes, Councils, and Statutes

**Abstract** The founding of Saint John hospital by burgher citizens and the role played by several lay members of the community, from the duke, to the castellan, to the aldermen, led to serious anxieties by the bishop of Cambrai. Fearing that he was losing control and concerned about heterodoxy, the bishop introduced a set of statutes to the hospital guaranteeing his position and assuring proper reform at the institution. This chapter considers why the bishop reasserted his power in the greater context of European affairs, namely the major ecumenical councils of Lateran III and Lateran IV, and the more regional French councils of the thirteenth century. As a result, the hospital became linked to important networks that in turn allowed the hospital to prosper before mid-century.

**Keywords** Burghers · Aldermen · Lateran III · Lateran IV · French Ecumenical Councils

## Introduction

As issues arose between the parish churches of Brussels and the hospital of Saint John, the Bishop of Cambrai, John of Bethune (r. 1200–1219 CE), was forced to mediate. The bishop's intervention into Saint John's

© The Author(s) 2018
T. A. Ziegler, *Medieval Healthcare and the Rise of Charitable Institutions*, The New Middle Ages, https://doi.org/10.1007/978-3-030-02056-9_6

affairs included providing the hospital with a set of statutes. Typically, regional hospitals received their statutes from bishops,[1] cathedral chapters, or more frequently from the priests, clergy, and aldermen of the city of the hospital's location.[2] The reception of the statutes not only made the hospital unique,[3] but also guaranteed the bishop's authority over the institution. According to the statutes, <u>secular authorities could not intervene</u>, while the Bishop of Cambrai held ultimate power in regard to matters of the hospital, especially the nomination of the *procureur*.[4] Also included in the hospital's statutes was the decree that the *procuerer* must have the consent of the bishop in certain matters.[5] This was a clear proclamation that authorities, such as the municipal figureheads of the castellan and duke, were not to intervene in the hospital's affairs. Moreover, the statutes reserved "no role for the prince, nor for the townsmen nor for the Brotherhood of the Holy Spirit to which the hospital owed its existence."[6]

In addition to demarking lines of intervention, the statutes also provided better organization for the growing hospital. The statutes allocated three brothers and ten sisters to run the hospital. The statutes also required the brothers and sisters to follow the Augustinian Rule; both men and women were to go through an examination period of four

---

[1] It was common for hospitals to be issued statutes by the local bishop. For more on this topic, see James Brodman, "Religion and Discipline in the Hospitals of Thirteenth-Century France," in *The Medieval Hospital and Medical Practice*, ed. Barbara Bowers (Burlington: Ashgate, 2007), 123–132. See especially page 126, where Bordman notes that of the twelve sets of statutes from 1162 to 1270, identified by Leon Le Grand in 1901, nine were issued "by the local bishop or his cathedral chapter."

[2] Bonenfant, *D'Histoire des Hôpitaux*, 27.

[3] "These [statutes] deserve special attention because of their uniqueness, their widespread influence, and the fact that they are among the oldest documents of this kind whose texts have been preserved. They seem quite original and cannot be connected with any of those which preceded them. On the contrary they became the prototype of those received by other hospitals of the diocese of Cambrai during the thirteenth and fourteenth centuries." Cherryhomes, "Charity in Brussels: The Hospital Saint John (1186–1300)," 77. It is also important to note that medicinal practices typically did not occur at similar institutions at this time, whereas they did at Saint John. Bonenfant, *D'Histoire des Hôpitaux*, 72.

[4] Bonenfant, *D'Histoire des Hôpitaux*, 28.

[5] *Cartulaire de l'Hôpital Saint-Jean*, SJ 10, p. 24. The original is lost. Later, Godfrey de Fontaines, bishop of Cambrai, approved the statutes again in 1225. See *Analectes pour servir à l'histoire ecclésiastique de la Belgique*, Vol. 29 (Louvain, 1901), 7.

[6] Cherryhomes, "Charity in Brussels: The Hospital Saint John (1186–1300)," 79.

months before being formally admitted into the community. The number of brothers and sisters remained small—thirteen—so that the personnel would not deplete the hospital funds and so that the institution would not grow to be big enough to become a monastery, which was not part of the original mission. Lay workers also assisted the hospital brethren with some of the domestic jobs. Once per week, the brothers and sisters met: one brother and one sister presided over the meetings and dealt out punishments according to infractions that had occurred.[7] Otherwise, the community was headed by a *procurator domus*, who was chosen from one of the brothers and who in turn formed part of the council of two of the other brothers—one being a priest—and four of the sisters.[8]

---

[7] This was normal and expected for a monastic community and thus proves to be a clear hold over from the early Middle Ages: "the community did correct the monks, but the monks described this discipline as stemming from their compassion and fraternal charity." See Martha G. Newman, *The Boundaries of Charity: Cistercian Culture and Ecclesiastical Reform, 1098–1180* (Stanford: Stanford University Press, 1996), 60–61.

[8] Bonenfant, *D'Histoire des Hôpitaux*, 27. The earliest known of the hospital masters was Brother Ludon (1230–1245). Later Masters Frédérick and Gautier also served as provisors. See *Cartulaire de l'Hôpital Saint-Jean*, SJ 205, 208, 219 regarding Frédérick; regarding Gautier see *Cartulaire de l'Hôpital Saint-Jean*, SJ 100, 101, 119, 122, 171, 172, 180, 191, 195, 197, 198, 200, 203, 204, 207, 210, 215, 216, 218, 222, 223, 224, 225, 226 227, 229, 241, 256, 266. Gautier was in both positions for a long time: 1257–1299. By the time we get to the end of our knowledge of him, he is being referred to as "*fratris Walteri de Sancto Johanne*." See *Cartulaire de l'Hôpital Saint-Jean*, SJ 266, pp. 321–322. CPAS SJ 45. The documents tend to note his different points of service. See charters 100 and 101 for a comparison. In charter 100, he is listed as "*fratri Waltero, provisori sancti ospitalis (sic) sancti Johannis in Bruxella*." *Cartulaire de l'Hôpital Saint-Jean*, SJ 100, pp. 138–139. CPAS SJ 38. In charter 101, he is simply listed as "*fratri Waltero*." *Cartulaire de l'Hôpital Saint-Jean*, SJ 101, pp. 139–140. CPAS SJ 29. At least two other brothers served the hospital: Godescalc (1298–1300; See *Cartulaire de l'Hôpital Saint-Jean*, SJ 249, 251, 253, 254, 259–264, 267, and 277) and Guillaume de Rodenbeke (1300): See *Cartulaire de l'Hôpital Saint-Jean*, SJ 270, 275, 276. Guilluame is a particularly hard character to pin down. He is not listed as master in document 270 or 275. Yet, document 276 has the name *magistro* on the back of the document. He may have been the brother to whom the document was referencing: "*Notum sit universis quod Franco de Papinghem promisit dare fratri Willelmo, dicto de Rodenbeke, fratri hospitalis beati Johannis in Bruxella...*". *Cartulaire de l'Hôpital Saint-Jean*, SJ 275, pp. 330–331. The original is lost. Finally, there were brothers who played administrative roles, such as Brother Gerard Carpentator. More likely than not, Gerard too was a master of the hospital. See *Cartulaire de l'Hôpital Saint-Jean*, SJ 121, 128, 131, 132, 139–145, 148, 151, 153, 164, 165, 188.

Although secular authorities, from the duke, to the townsmen, to the brothers of the confraternity, had all aided in its creation, it was made clear by the bishops that the hospital was to operate under religious expertise only, at least in the first half of the thirteenth century. The bishop's role in the institution thus placed the hospital on the same footing as the other religious houses in his dioceses, making the hospital exceptional in many regards.[9] Yet, the hospital was being treated like the monastic hospitals of the past—the religious community oversaw the bureaucracy of the hospital. This proved especially problematic in Brussels because of the explicit role of the secular townspeople in the founding of the institution, thereby placing the townspeople at odds with the local bishops.[10] Although embroiled in conflict, the debates between the religious and secular authorities made the hospital a success and made it unique: in the end, it became the first municipal hospital in Brussels. A deeper examination of the struggle is needed to fully comprehend the situation, for it is the struggle that created the municipal institution.

## THE STRUGGLE IS REAL: THE FIGHT BETWEEN CHURCH AND STATE

The struggle between religious and secular authorities in Brussels began even before the hospital was formed; in many ways, Saint John hospital was simply a microcosm of the greater issues occurring in Christendom. One of the first associates of the hospital was Bishop Roger de Wavrin (1178–1191 CE), who granted the confraternity of the Holy Spirit permission to form. Roger was an archdeacon and treasurer of Cambrai

---

[9] Brodman also explains that "there are other examples for Brussels, Tournai, Mons, and Lille," of which the statutes of the "Hospital of the Holy Spirit (St. John)" were important "because they were subsequently widely imitated in northern France." Brodman, *Charity and Religion*, 229.

[10] See Henne et Wauters, *Histoire de la Ville de Bruxelles*, 48–49. Also, Henry I was noted for his "munificence and piety" toward the hospital of Saint Jean. See H. De Bruyn, "Origine de l'Église et de l'hôpital de Saint-Jean, au Marais, a Bruxelles," in *Analectes Pour Servir à l'histoire ecclésiastique de la Belgique*, t. 4 (Brussels, 1867), 31. Over seven hundred years later, an 1846 inscription on the hospital honored this memory: "*a la pieuse et perpétuelle mémoire de Henri I, duc de Brabant, au fondateur et au plus grand bienfaiteure de l'Hôpital Saint-Jean.*" See *Administration Générale des Hospices et Secours de la ville de Bruxelles*. Hôpital Saint-Jean, from the collected material of CPAS, Brussels: Belgium, 7.

before taking the position of Bishop of Cambrai. He was consecrated in 1179 at Sainte-Sabine of l'Aventin by the Archbishop of Reims, Guillaume, who had been named cardinal by Pope Alexander III (1159–1181 CE) at Lateran III.[11] Roger had also participated in the Third Crusade with Raoul De Zähringen under the leadership of Frederick Barbarossa I (1123–1190 CE). Both men [Raoul and Roger] died in 1191 on the voyage back home—Roger died in the Holy Land itself while Raoul perished in Fribourg.

During Roger's period of service to the bishopric of Cambrai, Lateran III occurred. Lateran III,[12] called in 1179, is probably best known for ending the struggle between papacy and empire. Of particular importance here, however, are the canons that emerged from the council concerning the governance of the church, church offices, and other offices under the control of the church. The question of who had control over which sphere, religious or secular, was at the forefront. Town life in particular complicated a simple sacred and secular divide. The rise of popular piety further made matters more complex. A city like Brussels had clear secular rulers: the dukes and the castellans, and to some extent, the members of the town council. It also had clear religious rulers: priests, bishops, deacons, etc. What happens, though, in the case of a confraternity-turned-hospital? Both parties had been involved in its foundation; both parties wanted to see to its continued existence. The problem was, however, in the greater context of spiritual and secular struggles, shared governance was not possible, especially at a time when the church was flexing its muscles over secular leaders.

---

[11] Guillaume had been named a cardinal by Pope Alexander III (1159–1181) at Lateran III. S. J. É. de Moreau, *Histoire de l'église en Belgique*, 2ᵉ ed., t. III (Brussels, 1945), 76.

[12] The Third Lateran council was called by Pope Alexander (1159–1181) in 1178 and it was later held in Rome in March of 1179. We do not have the canons of this council, but we do have chronicles and annals that have preserved the acts of the council. See Abbot Benedict of Peterborough, Gervase of Canterbury, William of Newburgh, and Roger of Hoveden. *Decrees of the Ecumenical Councils*, ed. Norman P. Tanner (Washington, DC: Georgetown University Press, 1990). http://www.ewtn.com/library/COUNCILS/LATERAN3.HTM.

See also *Le Troisième Concile de Latran (1179): San place dans l'histoire*, Communications présentées à la Table Ronde du C.N.R.S. (Paris: Études Augustiniennes, 1982), 16, 51. The argument here suggests that the council was about progress via continuity.

The struggles of the church to reassert its power can be seen in Lateran III, canon nine, which reads, "Since we ought both to plant holy religion and in every way to cherish it when planted, we shall never fulfil this better than if we take care to nourish what is right and to correct what stands in the way of the progress of truth by means of authority entrusted to us."[13] Moreover, complaints had emerged regarding the Templars, Hospitallers, and other religious brotherhoods who were 'exceeding privileges' and 'disregarding episcopal authority',[14] while of grave concern was the admittance to those who were under the ban of excommunication and interdict to partake in the sacraments of the church. These same excommunicated peoples were granted burial.

In each of these cases, it was the circumvention of the church powers that was problematic, as many of the religious officials and groups were acting without the knowledge of the bishop, which in turned weakened the bishops' authority.[15] As a result, canon nine declared, regarding the brotherhoods,

> if any do not give themselves entirely to the said brothers but decide to keep their possessions, they are in no way on this account exempt from the sentence of the bishops, but the bishops may exercise their power over them as over other parishioners whenever they are to be collected for their faults. What has been said about the said brothers, we declare shall be observed with regard to other religious who presume to claim for themselves the rights of bishops and dare to violate their canonical decisions and the tenor of our privileges. If they do not observe this decree, let the churches in which they dare so to act be placed under an interdict, and let what they do be considered void.[16]

The significance of this passage lies in the clear attempt by the church to regain control over all matters related to its hierarchical governance of the church, including brotherhoods and hospitals. The formation of brotherhoods and hospitals challenged the authority of the church, and this was a way to solve that problem.

---

[13] *Decrees of the Ecumenical Councils*, ed. Norman P. Tanner, Lateran III, canon 9, http://www.ewtn.com/library/COUNCILS/LATERAN3.HTM.

[14] Ibid.

[15] Ibid.

[16] Ibid.

Another concern was the role of the laity in the matters of the church. Canon fourteen decreed that "since some of the laity have become so bold that disregarding the authority of bishops they appoint clerics to churches and even remove them when they wish, and distribute the property and other goods of the church for the most part according to their own wishes, and even dare to burden the churches themselves and their people with taxes and impositions, we decree that those who from now on are guilty of such conduct be punished by anathema."[17] Matters were explicitly to go through the channels of the church. This has already been noted with Saint John's and its statutes that dictated the absolute power of the bishop and the lack of outside secular power.

Moreover, episcopal authority over brotherhoods and hospitals was a way to enforce discipline. Between 1213 and 1215, several ecclesiastical councils were held in France, especially in Rouen and Paris. These councils were called to better prepare the church and reformers for upcoming Lateran IV, but also "affirmed the Church's responsibility over hospitals, particularly to ensure the honesty and propriety of their administration."[18] Among the concerns, fraud and abuse topped the list. Jacque de Vitry, a French bishop who praised Saint John hospital, was one of many bishops to note the abuses occurring at the so-called charitable institutions: "for under the pretext of hospitality and the guise of piety, they become alms collectors, improperly extorting monies by lies and deception and by every means at their disposal."[19] The bishops were genuinely concerned for the poor, and it is without a doubt that the reforming councils certainly influenced Saint John's statutes, which had provisions to help protect against fraud.[20]

The power of the church and the need for reform persisted with Lateran IV, called in 1215. Like Lateran III, Lateran IV continued to

[17] *Decrees of the Ecumenical Councils*, ed. Norman P. Tanner, Lateran III, canon 14, http://www.ewtn.com/library/COUNCILS/LATERAN3.HTM.

[18] James Brodman, "Religion and Discipline in the Hospitals of Thirteenth-Century France," in *The Medieval Hospital and Medical Practice*, ed. Barbara Bowers (Burlington: Ashgate, 2007), 125.

[19] Jacques de Vitry, *The Historia Occidentalis of Jacques de Vitry*, J. F. Hinnebusch, 148–149, cap. 29, in James Brodman, "Religion and Discipline in the Hospitals of Thirteenth-Century France," in *The Medieval Hospital and Medical Practice*, ed. Barbara Bowers (Burlington: Ashgate, 2007), 125.

[20] For more specific measures created to protect the institution from abuse, see the discussion of the statutes below.

assert and assure the power of the church. The sixth canon of Lateran IV, for example, specified that "the metropolitans must not neglect to hold with their suffragans the annual provincial synods."[21] Moreover, the canon instructed that "in reference to those things that they decree, let them enforce observance, publishing the decisions in the episcopal synods to be held annually in each diocese."[22] Canon fifty-seven granted "permission to some regulars that to those who have become members of their order, ecclesiastical burial may not be denied if the churches to which they belong should be under interdict, provided they themselves are not excommunicated or nominally interdicted; and they may, therefore, take their brethren, whom the prelates of the churches are not permitted to bury from their churches, to their own churches for burial, if they were not nominally under excommunication or interdict."[23] While the canon specifies 'the brethren', the idea behind the decree is that those who had given possessions to the institution via usufruct could be buried during interdict. This grant was widely applied to churches, monasteries, and even Saint John's hospital—not only could they bury during interdict, but they could also hold mass.[24]

---

[21] "Lateran IV, canon six," *Fordham Internet Sourcebook.* http://sourcebooks.fordham. edu/basis/lateran4.asp.

[22] Ibid.

[23] Ibid.

[24] During the dispute between the dean of Saint-Gudule and the hospital of Saint John, Pope Gregory IX granted to Saint John's hospital the ability to hold mass even when the doors were closed in times of interdict. *Cartulaire de l'Hôpital Saint-Jean,* SJ 38, 62. CPAS, SJ 4, fol. 5. The charter is damaged, but an analysis of the charter in 1589 provides the context of the bull. For that analysis, see *Cartulaire de l'Hôpital Saint-Jean,* 62. The prestige that followed in the wake of this privilege was augmented when on June 9, 1232 Pope Gregory IX extended his protection specifically to the prioress, the sisters, and their holdings. *Cartulaire de l'Hôpital Saint-Jean,* SJ 41, 66. CPAS, SJ 4. He repeated his extension of protection again on May 21, 1237. The brothers and the sisters of the hospital remained under his protection, as did the hospital and its holdings under his protection. *Cartulaire de l'Hôpital Saint-Jean,* SJ 50, 76. CPAS, SJ 4, fol. 7. Furthermore, the allowance suggests that there were cases in which the hospital might have been forced to close its doors. The local and international affairs of the dukes of Brabant and the bishop of Cambrai may have prompted this papal exemption, although it was a typical privilege that thirteenth-century popes often conferred. For information on the Dukes of Brabant, see de Moreau, *Histoire de l'église en Belgique;* Smets, *Henri I Duc de Brabant 1190–1235;* and Jean d'Anvers, *Brabantsche Yeesten,* J. F. Williams, *Les Gestes des Ducs de Brabant, par Jean de Klerk, D'Anvers* (Bruxelles, 1839). A second document granted the brothers and sisters of the hospital a priest and a cemetery. See *Cartulaire,* SJ 51, p. 77. The original is lost.

Between Lateran III and Lateran IV, Saint John hospital received its statutes[25] from Jean III, the Bishop of Cambrai, as noted above. Jean III of Béthune was consecrated in Rome, but owed his position to Otto IV (1175/6–1218 CE), as he was a supporter of Otto of Brunswick and Innocent III.[26] This not only linked the bishop of Cambrai to the struggle between the Empire and to the Papacy, but connected the hospital as well. More likely than not, Jean's good relationship with the papacy won the hospital its extension of papal protection.[27] Jean issued a second charter from Santbergen, a province in East Flanders, sometime between 7 and 30 April 1219, which remitted to the hospital of Saint John a portion of the tithes (*dîme*) of Leeuw-Saint-Pierre.[28] Bishop Jean III and eventually, Godfrey of Fontaines—the next bishop to have had a role in the hospital—found themselves engulfed in the papal–empire debate; both were forced to leave their positions because of the struggle.

---

[25] The importance of the statutes is profound. In 1963, Rawlins Cherryholmes argued that "these [statutes] deserve special attention because of their uniqueness, their widespread influence, and the fact that they are among the oldest documents of this kind whose texts have been preserved." Cherryholmes, "Charity in Brussels," 77. Only a few institutions and their statutes preceded Saint John Hospital: "the Hospital of Saint John of Jerusalem (between 1125 and 1153 and again in 1181), those of Aubrac (of 1162), and those of Montdidier (Somme) of 1207." Cherryholmes, "Charity in Brussels," 109.

[26] See Moreau, *Histoire de l'église en Belgique*, t. III, 161.

[27] It is also important to note that the charter mentions Duke Henry I: "*Henrici ducis Lotharingie munificentia et devotione.*" See Bonenfant, *Cartulaire de l'Hôpital Saint-Jean*, 19–25. See also Moreau, *Histoire de l'Église en Belgique*, t. I, 159–163, and t. III, 678.

[28] Today, Leeuw-Saint-Pierre is a small town on the outskirts of Brussels. It is sandwiched between Flanders and Belgium (it is in Flemish Brabant) and thus experiences ongoing problems related to language and nationality. Today, the official name of the commune is Sint-Pieters-Leeuw and the language principally spoken there is Dutch. "*...Presentium attestatione notum fieri volumes universis quod, honorabili viro Leonio, castellano Bruxellensi, a nobis postulante ut partem decime quam [ipse in] parrochia de Lewew possidebat de manu ejusdem recipient[tes] fratribus et sororibus hospitalis beati Johannis in Bruxella conferemus, nos eundem sedula ammonitione et exhotatione diligenti ad hoc studuimus inducer ut dictam decime portionem ad opus ecclesie illius resignaret ad cujus parrochiam pertinebat...*" *Cartulaire de l'Hôpital Saint-Jean*, SJ 14, p. 29. CPAS, SJ 40.

Godfrey of Fontaines (r. 1220–1237/38 CE),[29] the subsequent
bishop of Cambrai associated with the hospital, continued to support the
papacy even after the leaders involved changed to Frederick II (1194–
1250 CE) and Pope Honorius III (r. 1216–1227 CE). Godfrey was a
popular bishop and he was well known for his philanthropic acts.[30] On
June 15, 1220 at Soignies,[31] Godfrey confirmed an act that had been
issued sometime during the first half of that month by Hugues, the
abbot of Saint-Sépulcre of Cambrai from 1198 to 1221 that authorized the hospital of Saint John to purchase a *dîme* from Gui de Brages.[32]
Godfrey also reapproved the statutes of Saint John's hospital in 1220.[33]
In the meantime (1225–1226), Bishop Godfrey, Gautier, the dean
of Hal, Gautier de Braine, canon of Notre Dame of Cambrai, Raoul,
abbot of Ninove, and the knight Guillaume of Ledebergh were all working on a transfer of a chapel in Ledebergh in the parish of Pamele[34] to
the hospital of Saint John.[35] The chapel would eventually provide the
hospital with a priest.[36] The relationship with the papacy once again

[29] De Moreau, *Histoire de l'Église en Belgique*, t. III, 164. While Godfrey was the only
bishop to issue four documents pertaining to the hospital (23.5% of the documents issued
by bishops and 1.4% of the total of all the documents), Godfrey's role was more reserved.
Godfrey was just as embroiled in struggle against the commune as his predecessor Jean III.
He was even forced in 1223 to leave his bishopric as Jean III did. As the battles between
the papacy and the empire also continued with Frederick II and Pope Honorius III (1216–
1227), so did Godfrey's role in the affairs, which may have limited or even dictated the
ways in which Godfrey responded to the hospital.

[30] De Moreau, *Histoire de l'Église en Belgique*, t. III, 166. De Moreau alludes to the fact
that Godfrey was known for charitable acts, but he provides no other elaboration on the
subject before moving on to the next bishop. It seems that the evidence for his charity can
be verified in the charters of the hospital of Saint Jean.

[31] Soignies is located outside of Brussels.

[32] "...*Presentium testimonio notum facimus universis quod hospitali beati Johannis in
Bruxella indulsimus quod decimam, quam in parrochia nostra de Tornepia Wido de Birthe
et Nicholaus, fratres, et Reinekinus possederunt, comparare posset. Hac adjecta conditione
quod quandocumque voluerimus eandem nobis redimere, licebimus, dum modo summam pecu-
nie, qua decimam predictam a memoratis comparaverit, eidem hospitali persolverimus...*"
*Cartulaire de l'Hôpital Saint-Jean*, SJ 15, pp. 31–32. CPAS, SJ 45.

[33] See *Cartulaire de l'Hôpital Saint-Jean*, SJ 20, p. 38. The original has been lost.

[34] *...Pamellam in capella de Ledeberghe.* See Bonenfant, *Cartulaire de l'Hôpital Saint-
Jean*, 48.

[35] *Cartulaire de l'Hôpital Saint-Jean*, SJ 49, pp. 75–76. The original is lost.

[36] For more on the hospital chapel, see De Bruyn, "Origine de l'Église et de l'hôpital de
Saint-Jean, au Marais, a Bruxelles."

brought support to the hospital during Godfrey's stint as bishop, as Pope Honorius III (r. 1216–1227 CE) extended his protection over the hospital once on October 28, 1218, once on April 27, 1219, and a third time on December 2, 1225. The first charter was issued from Lateran, the second from Rome, and the third from Rieti.

Later, Pope Gregory IX (r. 1227–1241 CE) followed suit by granting Saint John hospital the ability to hold mass even during periods of interdict in 1231. Gregory IX extended his protection over the hospital in 1232, and finally, on May 27, 1237, he reconfirmed his protection of the hospital and its ability to remain open even during periods of interdict.[37] Working closely with the Bishop of Cambrai, Godfrey, Pope Gregory IX allowed the bishop of Cambrai to grant the hospital a priest and cemetery. Clearly, there was a relationship between pope, bishop, and hospital.

Bishop Godfrey also confirmed the statutes of Saint John's hospital that had been granted under his precursor that same year (1220),[38] going as far as to rededicate the statues in honor of his predecessor.[39] He again reconfirmed the statutes in 1225.[40] On January 27, 1225, Godfrey, the Bishop of Cambrai, "delegated his powers to Gautier, dean of Hal canon of Cambrai, for the erection of the *chapellenie* that Guillaume de Ledeberg, knight, wanted to establish at the hospital of Saint Jean."[41] In October 1236, Godfrey approved the transfer of the office of the *chapellenie* of Ledebergh.[42]

---

[37] See above regarding Lateran III and IV.

[38] For explanation on the date, see Bonenfant, notes to the act, *Cartulaire de l'Hôpital Saint-Jean*, SJ 20, p. 37.

[39] *Quoniam injuncti nobis officii est a predecessoribus nostris salubriter inchoate ad consummationis bonum perducere, que felicis memorie predecessoris nostril domini Johannis, quondam Cameracensis episcope, auctoritate, de prudentium virorum consilio* and *Sicut igitur memoriati pontificis prudencia et devocione observancie regulars n hopstiali beati Johannis in Bruxella regulariter sunt institute, sic easdem scripti presentis duximus approbatione confrimandas.* See *Cartulaire de l'Hôpital Saint-Jean*, SJ 20, p. 38. The original has been lost.

[40] See *Analectes pour servir à l'histoire ecclésiastique de la Belgique*, Vol. 29 (Louvain, 1901), 7.

[41] "*G., Dei gratia Cameracensis episcopus, viro venerabili et dilecto in Christo G., decano de Hal, canonico Cameracensi, salute et sinceram dilectionem. Intelleximus quod vir nobilis Willelmus de Ledeberga miles, in domo hospitalis sancti Johannis in Bruxella pro sua et antecessorum suorum salute perpetuam vult instituere capellaniam de bonis suis, quam petit auctoriate nostra dicte domui confirmari.*" See *Cartulaire de l'Hôpital Saint-Jean*, SJ 23, pp. 41–42.

[42] *Cartulaire de l'Hôpital Saint-Jean*, SJ 49, pp. 75–76. The original is lost.

Gui I (Gui or Guiard de Laon r. 1237–1247 CE)[43] was the next bishop of Cambrai.[44] The first charter he issued was on December 22, 1240 and was in direct relation to a previous papal bull that had been issued by Pope Gregory IX on May 22, 1237.[45] In the bull, Pope Gregory IX had allowed the Bishop of Cambrai to grant a priest and a cemetery to the brothers and sisters of the hospital of Saint John. In 1240, the privilege was again reevaluated, this time by Bishop Gui who reconfirmed Gregory IX's allowances to the hospital of Saint John. The brothers and sisters were to receive the cemetery[46] on the occasion of the funeral of Jacques, the son of Guillaume of Ledebergh.[47] Gui I passed the responsibility to the dean of chapter of Sainte-Gudule,[48] under whose intervention the hospital of Saint John had originally been placed. A second charter issued by Bishop Gui I occurred on September 17, 1242 when Gui I made it known to the rural dean[49] of Sainte-Gudule that he was revoking a previous ruling that was burdening both the

---

[43] Gui is identified as Guiard de Laon by Bonenfant. See Bonenfant, *Cartulaire de l'Hôpital Saint-Jean*, SJ 55, p. 82, fn I.

[44] Moreau, *Histoire de l'Église en Belgique*, t. III, 166.

[45] See above. *Cartulaire de l'Hôpital Saint-Jean*, SJ 51, p. 77.

[46] "…*Inde est quod vobis mandamus quatenus, ad decanum et capitulum Bruxellense personaliter accedentes, ipsos ex parte nostra moneatis, rogantes eosdem ut permittant predictis fratribus corpora fratrum et sororum ac pauperum, qui in dicta domo decesserint, in cimiterio, quod habere dicuntur, sepelire nec impediant quominus illi qui elegerint in dicta domo sepulturam, sive sint parochiani sancte Gudule sive alterius parochie, ibidem valeant sepeliri, precipue cum dicti fraters, sicut nobis ex parte eorum intimatum est, parati sint et fuerint quoslibet conservare indempnes super jure sepulture predictorum et aliis quibuscumque…*" *Cartulaire de l'Hôpital Saint-Jean*, SJ 55, p. 82. The original is lost.

[47] "…*Verum, cum nuper sicut intelleximus, dicti decanus et capitulum corpus cujusdam Jacobi defunct, filii quodam Willielmi de Ledeberghe, qui Jacobus in neadem domo habitum eorum susceperat et decesseit, in prejudicium dictorum fratrum non modicum et gravamen ab eadem domo asportaverint violenter, ita quod dicti fraters corpus ipsius non potuerint ecclesiastice trader sepulture, vobis iterate mandamus, quatenus dictos decanum et capitulum moneatis ut, si ita est, super hoc dictis fratribus satisfaciant indilate, alioquin dictis fratribus deesse non poterimus, quin secundum mandatum apostolicum ipsis exhibeamus juris debiti complementum…*" *Cartulaire de l'Hôpital Saint-Jean*, SJ 55, p. 82.

[48] *Cartulaire de l'Hôpital Saint-Jean*, SJ 55, p. 82.

[49] "*G., Dei gratia Cameracensis episcopus, dilecto filio plebano Bruxellensi…*" *Cartulaire de l'Hôpital Saint-Jean*, SJ 60, p. 87.

brothers and sisters of the hospital of Saint John and preventing them from delivering their goods and services.[50]

With the creation of the chapel, the protection of the papacy, the reception of a priest, and the ability to have a cemetery, involvement from other religious institutions continued to increase. On October 10, 1241, the tenth abbot of Afflighem (r. 1227–1242), Guillaume, approved a sale that had been made between the hospital of Saint John and Henry, the chaplain of the monastery.[51] The sale included two *bonniers* (*duobus bonariis*) of land located in the parish of Assche. Eight years later, in August 1249, Abbot Daniel and the monastery of Grimbergh sold the hospital a portion of arable lands that they held in allodium in the parish of Cortenbergh,[52] and in July 1253, the abbess of the convent of Forest approved a transfer of land in Anderlecht near Ransfort made to the hospital of Saint John.[53]

At each point illuminated here, the bishops were making their authority in the hospital known. It seems that their intentions were met with success. From a flexing of church muscle, however, came the ideal example of a municipal hospital. Saint John hospital not only flourished in the mid-thirteenth century thanks to the intervention of the bishops, but it became a model to which other hospitals looked.

---

[50] "...*Cum apostolus ad ipsum pertingere asserat infirmitates quorumlibet aliorum, terror nobis incutitur si, quorum cura nobis committitur, utputa hospitalium et ibidem egrotancium, quorum disposition et defensio nostro incumbit officio, eorum paci et tranquillitati providere negligamus. Ne igitur servitutibus in rebus propriis aggraventur qui defectu virium, paupertate et egritudine opprimuntur, volumes et decernimus ne qlique servitudes in rebus suis, vie, itineris, usus vel usufructus, a rectoribus hospitalis sancti Johannis in Bruxella in nostra diocese constitute, fratribus vel sororibus ejusdem hospitalis, cuiquam concedatur (sic.). Quod si contra fecerint, id irritum habeatur et tam dans quam recipiens indignationem Domini incurrere vereatur. Ad quod exequendum, scilicet quod in hac parte statuimus, te exequtorem deputamus, mandates tibi quatinus quicquid in hac parte contra hoc inveneris attemptari in statum pristinum revokes, attemptantes ad desistendum per censuram ecclesiasticam compellendo, ut sic libertate rerum suarum dictum hospitale ab inquietudine que exinde posset contingere defenduatur...*" Cartulaire de l'Hôpital Saint-Jean, SJ 60, pp. 87–88. CPAS, SJ 4.

[51] *Cartulaire de l'Hôpital Saint-Jean*, SJ 56, pp. 82–83. CPAS, SJ 35, fol. 49.

[52] *Cartulaire de l'Hôpital Saint-Jean*, SJ 76, pp. 112–113. CPAS, SJ 36, fol. 56.

[53] *Cartulaire de l'Hôpital Saint-Jean*, SJ 85, pp. 122–123. CPAS, SJ 36, fol. 20.

## BEYOND THE HOSPITAL PROPER: THE APPEAL OF ITS STATUTES

From 1211 to 1253, the bishops of Cambrai and the papacy became increasingly involved with the affairs of Saint John hospital in Brussels. The amount of attention that the hospital received from these figures deserves a deeper examination. Indeed, the biggest question that remains is, why? Why this hospital? Before Saint John hospital in Brussels, the statutes of the hospitals throughout Europe and beyond were varied and inconsistent. Aubrac and Angers hospitals, for example, were both founded before Saint John in Brussels; however, Aubrac's statutes were quite short, while those of Angers were rather long. Other hospitals, such as the Hôtel-Dieu at Amiens and Montdidier, had statutes that proved to be more consistent and as a result were subsequently applied to Maisons Dieu in Noyon (1218) and others (1234).[54]

The statutes of Saint John hospital begin with a brief introduction, which identifies the Bishop of Cambrai, John, the hospital, and the Duke of Brabant, Henry I. Thirty-six rules then follow. The majority of the rules instruct the brothers and sisters how to act and live: the brothers and sisters were to live and dress with modesty (1); no feather mattresses were allowed unless you were sick (4); brothers and sisters were not to wear linen underneath their woolen habits (5); brothers and sisters were to remain in separate dorms, refectories, and offices of administration (6); brothers and sisters were to maintain silence after dinner (14); one time per week, a priest was to bring the group together to discuss incidents (15); and finally, a long list of days as to when to fast were outlined (17).

It is only in the latter half of the statutes that the care of the sick is outlined along with medical care that they were to receive. The statutes make it clear that care is for those who are poor and those who are too sick to beg (22). In addition, when the sick entered into the hospital, they had to confess their sins and do works of satisfaction (23). If it was necessary, a physician could be called in particular instances (25).

---

[54] Léon Le Grand, *Statuts d'hotels-Dieu et de léproseries; recueil de textes du XII<sup>e</sup> au XIV<sup>e</sup> siècle* (Paris: Alphonse Picard et Fils, 1901), 34. According to Brodman, the collection published by Leon Le Grand, "contains the statutes of a dozen municipal hospitals and another thirteen leprosaries. The earliest and simplest cited text is that of the Pyrenean Hospital of Aubrac, dating from 1162. Another eleven date from about 1200 to 1270; of these, nine were issued by the local bishop or his cathedral chapter, one by a local count, and another." Brodman, *Charity and Religion*, 229.

The most defining regulations, however, are numbers twenty six and seven: pregnant women without family or homes were to be received to give birth and were able to stay at the hospital until they were capable of providing for the child (26), while any orphans left to the hospital were to be cared for by the hospital staff where medical care was clearly provided. The remainder of the rules dealt with prayers for the dead and the role of the bishop in all matters.[55]

The statutes of the hospital of Saint John in Brussels produced consistency while attributing action to an embodiment of *caritas*. Interestingly, the uniformity lies in the mission as originally prescribed by the confraternity of the Holy Spirit and its patrons: care for the poor, but also the sick, infants, orphans, and pregnant women. This idea was innovative and Saint John hospital in Brussels was at the core of its creation. It merged the monastic hospital movement and the lay charity movement while also enforcing the reforms as dictated by the French reforming councils. The hospital of Saint John's statutes subsequently became the model for hospitals of the diocese of Cambrai and beyond throughout the thirteenth and fourteenth centuries.[56] Other institutions as far away as the Hôtel-Dieu of Paris also modeled their statutes after the hospital of Saint John.[57] In all, the following institutions modeled their statutes on the hospital of Saint John:

- Notre-Dame de Cambrai (probably before 1220)
- Hôtel-Dieu Saint-Julien of Cambrai (probably before 1220)
- The Hôtel-Dieu of Paris in 1220 (other dates suggest between 1217 and 1221)
- The Hospital of Notre-Dame in Anvers (1233)
- The Hospital of Hérenthals in October 1253

---

[55] *Cartulaire de l'Hôpital Saint-Jean*, SJ 10, pp. 19–25. The original is lost.

[56] Bonenfant, *Cartulaire de l'Hôpital Saint-Jean*, XVII.

[57] Of special note in this list is the Hôtel-Dieu of Paris, which was, by this point, about five times the size of Saint John. The hospital at Paris received its statutes between 1217 and 1221 and imitated those of Saint John. Shortly after Paris received its statutes, Jacques de Vitry named the Hospital of Saint John of Brussels as one of the greatest hospitals of its time, numbering it among hospitals like the Hôtel-Dieu of Paris. The connection between Paris, Jacques, and the reform councils seems evident. The Hôtel-Dieu of Paris probably in wake of the reforms of the 1213 and 1214 councils sought out a set of statutes that best met the issues raised at the councils. The fact that Paris chose to imitate Saint John speaks to the quality and importance of the statutes.

- The Hospital of Sainte-Gudule of Brussels (the previous hospital of Notre-Dame and the Twelve Apostles) in February 1256
- The Hospital of Gheel in August 1284
- The Leprosarium of Saint Pierre in Brussels in 1220 (Godfrey of Fontaine)
- The Hospital of Notre-Dame de Malines (Godfrey of Fontaine)
- The Hospital Notre-Dame à la Rose of Lessines (Bishop Gui de Laon) in 1247
- The Hospital of Notre-Dame of Grammont in 1255
- The Hospital of Alost in 1266
- The Hospital of Merchtem in the fourteenth century
- The Hospital in Mons
- The Hospital in Lille[58]

What, exactly, was going on? In a simple answer, these people—popes, bishops, priests, hospital brothers and sisters—were all part of an inner circle that communicated with each other in order to reform and control all laic institutions, hospitals included. It was, in some ways, a reassertion of power that the church had once had in its early years. Yet, exchange and interaction did not end with the bishops. The hospital corresponded with priests, clerics, brothers, deans, abbots, abbesses, and canons associated with or from the cities of Anvers, Forest, Grimbergh, Louvain, Jette, Alost, Affligem, Meerbeke, Ninove, Hal, Nivelles, Cortenbergh, Anderlecht, Scripburg, Strythem, Pede, Hartbeke, Drootbeek, Soignies, Pamele, Cambrai, Meerbeek, Gysegem (in East Flanders), Laeken, Machelen, Linkebeek, Auderghem, Ledebergh, and Tournai. The masters and administrators of Saint John hospital also exchanged communication with popes Innocent III, Honorius III, and Gregory IX, and legates (Pierre Capocci—Alexander IV) at Montefiascone, Santbergen, the Lateran, Rome, Rieti, Spolète, and Viterbe. A network existed along which information was disseminated and exchanged, including the statutes of the hospital of Saint John, to best meet the growing needs of the hospital movement.

---

[58] Mons and Lille have been identified by Brodman. The rest were first named by Bonenfant.

## CONCLUSION

The hospital of Saint John in Brussels was not the first nor only hospital of the high Middle Ages. Other hospitals rose rapidly in this period from Girona to Avignon.[59] Yet, the hospital of Saint John in Brussels serves as an example of how hospitals in this period arose from complicated struggles between the clergy and the townsmen. Although the hospital did not play a role per se in that greater Empire–Church struggle, it did benefit from the repercussions of association. The intervention by the bishop in 1211, which provided the hospital of Saint John with its statutes, set in motion a chain of events. The new statutes combined the older traditions of the monastic hospital with the newer mission of the Peace of God movements, such as that of the confraternity of the Holy Spirit. The statutes of Saint John hospital were then disseminated along the networks of the greater area and subsequently applied to other hospitals. The initial vying for power by the dukes, the town castellan, the burgher class, and the bishops resulted in the creation of the city's first municipal hospital. This is made even more apparent in the events that followed when the burgher citizens resumed a significant role in the institution's direction and management.

---

[59]For a fuller and varied list of the many institutions that appeared in this period, see James Brodman, *Charity and Religion*.

# PART III

# The Birth of the Municipal Hospital

# CHAPTER 7

# The Rise of Brussels' Municipal Hospital

**Abstract** The hospital of Saint John in Brussels remains important for two pivotal reasons: its statutes and its continued involvement by the people of the town. This chapter considers what occurred at the hospital of Saint John after its creation and after the dissemination of its statutes. Mid century saw an indulgence campaign that allowed for the hospital to rebuild. Primary in the campaign was the concept of *Amor civicus*; the peoples of Brussels donated money and lands to the reconstruction of their beloved hospital. By 1300, Saint John hospital was Brussels' first true municipal hospital.

**Keywords** Donations · Patrons · Burghers · Aldermen · Brussels · Urbanization · Public

## INTRODUCTION

The hospital, especially in the second half of the thirteenth century, grew exponentially, thanks to generous patrons: it "inherited the possessions of the sick who died intestate; those who left wills could give away only the part of their possessions in excess of the cost of care at the hospital; but in the case of recovery, the hospital demanded nothing."[1] Initially, the hospital

---

[1] Marx, *The Development of Charity in Medieval Louvain*, 36.

© The Author(s) 2018
T. A. Ziegler, *Medieval Healthcare and the Rise of Charitable Institutions*, The New Middle Ages, https://doi.org/10.1007/978-3-030-02056-9_7

brothers supervised the grants that were provided to the hospital. Later, a board of lay advisors, or provisors, saw to the interest of the hospital.[2] The lay advisors were drawn from the same offices as the original brothers of the confraternity. Moreover, these were the same peoples from which the office of the magistrate were drawn, the *échevins*, by the middle of the thirteenth century, the office of the provisors was that of the *échevins*, thus merging the two. Although bearing the burden of the hospital's administration could be seen as a negative, the fact that the city continued to administer the hospital up through the modern period speaks to the institution's importance. It becomes clear through a brief examination of the hospital's early history that the institution was a matter of concern for multiple parties in the city of Brussels. The question remained, however, who would ultimately govern the hospital: public or private entities or both?

## THE RETURN OF THE BURGHER CLASS

On August 27, 1254, Pierre Capocci, a cardinal legate, accorded thirty days of indulgences to those who made donations to the mistress, the brothers, or the sisters[3] for the reconstruction of the hospital,[4] which apparently was in need of repair by mid century. The indulgence campaign and the creation of a new facility may have instigated greater outside involvement. The bull describes the hospital as having been newly planted[5] and offers indulgences to those who would help in its construction.[6]

---

[2] Paul Evrard has addressed the lessening involvement of the papacy and the increased involvement of the papacy in Paul Evrard, "Formation, organization, générale et état du domaine rural de l'hôpital Saint-Jean au Moyen-Âge," 7. In addition, I have also argued for the increased role of the aldermen in hospital affairs, which too negated the need for the bishops. These two aspects, however, cannot be separated as many of the provisors were also aldermen. See Tiffany A. Ziegler, "Considering Networks of Charity: Family Traditions, Female Donation Practices, and the Hospital of Saint John's in Brussels," *The Journal of Medieval Prosopography*, Vol. 29 (2015).

[3] *Cartulaire de l'Hôpital Saint-Jean*, SJ 91, p. 130. CPAS, SJ 4, fol. 18.

[4] Ibid.

[5] ... *quod est novella plantation*. CPAS, SJ 4, fol. 18.

[6] ... *inceperint edificare de novo opera sumptuous*. CPAS, SJ 4, fol. 18. Meredith Parsons Lillich has made some commentary on the future perfect uses of the word *inceperint*. See Meredith Parsons Lillich, "The Choir Clerestory Windows of La Trinité at Vendôme: Dating and Patronage," *The Journal of the Society of Architectural Historians*, Vol. 34, No. 3 (October 1975), pp. 238–250 and specifically 244–245.

Gradually, the old hospital buildings were renovated, during which time the sisters, headed by a prioress (*magistra*), took on more administrative duties. The mistress oversaw the community, whereas the brothers were in charge of the administration of the holdings.[7] There is a clear break in those active in the hospital and its administration. From its creation to 1211, the concern of the hospital was limited greatly to local authorities. After 1211, the bishops of Cambrai played an increasingly important role, up through the 1240s. In fact, between 1231 and 1240, only one document was issued by the aldermen's court. Four more documents were issued from the aldermen's court between 1241 and 1250 and another four from 1251 to 1260. In the 1240s, 1250s, and 1260s, there are fewer appearances—the bishops subsequently started to decline while the aldermen started to play an increased role. By 1300, the hospital was under clear secular control. The following illustrates how rapidly the aldermen's court appeared after 1260:

- 1231–1240: 1 act—bishops still in control
- 1241–1250: 4 acts—rebuilding
- 1251–1260: 4 acts—rebuilding
- 1261–1270: 26 acts
- 1271–1280: 22 acts
- 1281–1290: 22 acts
- 1291–1300: 39 acts[8]

The simple equation that giving and providing equaled salvation created a new-found success for charity and healthcare, the "clearest proof of [which was] the widespread popular support their hospitals immediately attracted."[9] Popular support at the hospital of Saint John could not be more apparent. From its inception, the burgher class worked to assure the confraternity's success. Then, throughout the hospital's thirteenth century history, numerous burghers appear in the records, some of the most frequent of which were Arken, Beatrix, Boete, Clabot, Eggloy, Molenbeek, Platea, Roede, Rulin, Scipburg, Spieghel. At times, these

---

[7] This change of roles by the brothers and sisters has been already noted in historical scholarship. Cherryhomes, "Charity in Brussels: The Hospital Saint John (1186–1300)," 78.

[8] Bonenfant, *Cartulaire de l'Hôpital Saint-Jean*, XLVIII.

[9] Kealey, *Medieval Medicus*, 83.

burghers played the supporting role of alderman, witness, provisor, and so forth. At other times, they provided donations to the hospital. The family members of the original burghers also went on to patronize the hospital.[10]

Yet, after the construction of the new hospital buildings, the breadth of peoples associated with the hospital expanded considerably. The hospital became *the* place to donate. A quick survey of the extant documents reveals that following peoples made donations: miller, butcher, hangman, candle maker, cobblers, alderman, justices, clerics, secretary, fisherman, weaver, blacksmith, notaries, a doctor of theology, farmers, chroniclers, cloth dyers, scholars, and more. And why not? It was the only institution other than the leprosarium of Saint Pierre to care for the public. It was the only institution open for general care.[11] These very peoples also saw the poor and sick recently brought into view by the effects of urbanization. Viewing those less fortunate, while being casually reminded of the place that could help the sick, prompted Brussels' inhabitants to provide graciously to the hospital of Saint John in a fashion that can only be described as centralized.

In approximately twenty-five years, the hospital went from a private confraternity and retiree community to a centralized general hospital. Its statutes specified the care that was to be given to pregnant women and orphaned children, to those too ill to beg and to those too sick to care for themselves. This was no longer a private hospital: it was a centralized public one that existed thanks to private donations. Caring was for all by all. It is thus without surprise that the hospital increased in size and renown throughout the 1200s.

## CONCLUSION

In 1294, Jean II took over as duke of Brabant,[12] and the original role of the dukes of Brabant in the hospital continued under him. In addition, Bishop Gui II de Colmieu served as a bishop of Cambrai from 1296 to

---

[10] See Tiffany A. Ziegler, "Considering Networks of Charity: Family Traditions, Female Donation Practices, and the Hospital of Saint John's in Brussels," *The Journal of Medieval Prosopography*, Vol. 29 (2015).

[11] The care given and who received care was described in the statutes as noted above.

[12] Jean the Peaceful. Was the son of Jean I; worked to stop French expansion.

1306; he too made a reappearance at the institution.[13] The last three charters of bishops were all issued by him.[14] In January 1300, Jean II granted the hospital lands held in census to him.[15] In February 1300, the Duke of Brabant, Jean II referred to Saint John hospital as *"hospitalis noster:"*[16] ad opus hospitalis nostri sancti Johannis in Bruxella et non alicujus alterius."[17] The emphatic, "not to any other" is key. Finally, on March 25, 1300 Bishop Gui II allowed the hospital of Saint John to establish a new cemetery.[18]

---

[13] Bonenfant, *Cartulaire de l'Hôpital Saint-Jean*, 304, fn 3.

[14] Gui II was named to the bishopric of Cambrai by Boniface VIII. So where influenced by the popes may seem to drop off after John XXI, it does continue, but only indirectly. See de Moreau, *Histoire de l'Église en Belgique*, t. III, 210. His 8 April 1298 charter approved and confirmed the indulgences that were granted by the group of bishops, archbishops and patriarchs mentioned in the previous issuance "...*confectas pro hospitale beati Johannis in Bruxella, nostre diocesis, et earum inspecto tenore, quia opus pietatis existit sanctorum limina visitare ac ecclesiis et pauperibus subvenire, quidquid per ipsos archiepiscopos et episcopos actum est in hac parte ratum et firmum habemus et illud, prout in ipsis exprimitur litteris, omnibus vere penitentibus et confessis auctoritate ordinaria cum quadraginta dierum indulgentiss confirmamus...*" *Cartulaire de l'Hôpital Saint-Jean*, SJ 250, pp. 304–305. The original is lost. "...*Ex parte vestra fuit nobis humiliter supplicatum, quod, cum vestry hospitalis cimiterium sit adeo corporum defunctorum repletum quod, cum vestri hospitalis cimiterium sit adeo corporum defunctorum repletum quod ibidem pro decedentibus christianis sepeliendis nequitis vacuum invenire, ut cimiterium alud decicandi ad opus hospitalis ejusdem concedere licentiam dignaremur. Nos vero, volentes vestries piis petitionibus complacere, construendi et edificandi aliud cimiterium sine alterius prejudicio, in honesto tamen loco, ac ab aliquot catholico episcopo ecclesie Romane devote dedicandi et benedictionem impendendi, auctoritate presentium, de speciali gratia vobis plenam concedimus potestatem...*" *Cartulaire de l'Hôpital Saint-Jean*, SJ 271, p. 326. Gui also authorized on 25 March 1300 at Thun-l'Évêque the establishment of a new cemetery for the hospital of Saint John since its previous cemetery had been filled. Finally, on 10 September 1300 Gui issued a charter that would allow the master, brothers, the mistress and the sisters of the hospital of Saint Jean to consume milk, cheese, eggs and butter during Advent, and to likewise be able to wear shoes of leather. "...*Pio vobis paterno compatientes affect, vobis tenore presentium indulgemus et de gratia speciali concedimus ut de ceteris in quolibet Adventu Domini album esum, silicet (sic) lac, caseum, ova et butirum, commedere licere[t] ac suttellares seu calciamenta de corduano ad usum vestrum et utilitatem deferre et ut auctoritate nostra possitis, aliqua nostrum presentibus est appensum...*" *Cartulaire de l'Hôpital Saint-Jean*, SJ 276, pp. 331–332. CPAS, SJ 5.

[15] *Cartulaire de l'Hôpital Saint-Jean*, SJ 269, pp. 324–325. CPAS, SJ 37.

[16] *Cartulaire de l'Hôpital Saint-Jean*, SJ 269, p. 325. CPAS, SJ 37.

[17] Ibid.

[18] *Cartulaire de l'Hôpital Saint-Jean*, SJ 271, pp. 326–327. The original is lost.

Overall, the importance of the hospital is paramount. By far, Saint John's hospital was, at least in the thirteenth century, one of the largest and most important hospitals in Europe at this time. Contemporary Jacques de Vitry ranked it along with the Hôtels-Dieu of Paris, of Noyon, of Provins, of Tournai and of Liège.[19] It was *the* municipal hospital of Brussels, and as a public building it "expressed the ambitions and ideology of a collectivity, the organized community of town citizens itself, of the craft guilds, and other corporate bodies (fraternities, shooting guilds, rhetoricians)."[20] Yet, little attention has been given to it. While its survival well into the early modern era attests to its local success, it found great notoriety beyond Brussels; Saint John's statutes served as a model for other hospitals, such as those in Antwerp, Mechelen, and Liège.

Today, only reflections of the hospital remain. The Rue de l'Hôptial is a very old road that links the Place of Saint John with the Place of Justice.[21] Before becoming Rue de l'Hôptial, it was called the Rue du Marquis and had three important buildings during the Middle Ages: the hôtel des barons de Thysebaert and three hospitals/hospices: Sainte-Gudule, la Trinité and Calvaire.[22] Currently, the north side borders the former hospital of Saint John. The hospital survived until 1843, at which time the sick were transferred to a new Hospital of Saint John on the boulevard du Jardin Botanique. The old hospital was destroyed in 1846 along with the church.[23] Saint Jean Place is where a number of streets

---

[19] Cherryholmes, "Charity in Brussels: The Hospital Saint John (1186–1300)," 71. See also *Cartulaire*, VIII, and the *Historia Occidentalis* of Jacques de Vitry: "Parisiis autem in Nouiomi in Francia, Pruuini in Campania et Tornaci in Flandria et Leodii in Lotharingia et Bruscellis in Brabantia, sunt hospitalia pietatis et domus honestatis, officine sanctitatis, conuentus decoris et religionis, refugia pauperum, auxilium miserorum, consolations lugentium, refection esurientium, suauitas et mitigation infirmorum." John Frederick Hinnebusch, *The Historia Occidentalis of Jacques de Vitry: A Critical Edition* (Fribourg: The University Press, 1972), 150–151.

[20] Peter Stabel, "The Marketplace and Civic Identity in Late Medieval Flanders" in *Shaping Urban Identity in Late Medieval Europe*, eds. Marc Boone and Peter Stabel (Leuven-Apeldoorn: Garant, 2000), 52.

[21] Jean d'Osta, *Dictionnaire historique et anecdotique des Rues de Bruxelles* (Bruxelles: Paul Legrain, 1986), 149.

[22] Jean d'Osta, *Les rues disparues de Bruxelles* (Rossel: Belgique, 1979), 86.

[23] Jean d'Osta, *Dictionnaire historique et anecdotique des Rues de Bruxelles*, 149.

converge: Lombard, de la Violette, des Eperonniers, Duqesnoy, Saint-Jean, de l'Hôpital, and l'amorce de la Vieille Hall aux Blés. It is not an old area; constructed between 1845 and 1846 at the same time as the rues of Dusquesnoy and Saint John.[24] Although the building is gone, the memory of the hospital remains.

[24] Jean d'Osta, *Dictionnaire historique et anecdotique des Rues de Bruxelles*, 305.

# CHAPTER 8

# Conclusion

**Abstract** The history of the municipal hospital is long and complicated. Although the rise of the municipal hospital occurred in the Middle Ages, the traditions that created the institution began long before the medieval period. While it might seem senseless to reinvent the wheel, or in this case the hospital, the overall history of the hospital is key in understanding its ultimate development. The history of the hospital is not one of only the institutional building; it is the history of the people associated with the hospital and its creation. In the conclusion, we revisit the rise of the hospital from its primitive stages to the rise of medieval hospital of Saint John in order to understand the importance of these transitions today.

**Keywords** Municipal hospital · Middle Ages · Saint John hospital · Healthcare

## EARLY CARE AND INSTITUTIONS

The earliest care provided to peoples who were sick and injured did not occur within the confines of a formal building. Ancient healers simply applied techniques of washing, bandaging, and setting bones on an ad hoc basis wherever the care was needed. The rise of 'civilizations' changed the ways in which healthcare was provided. Centralized

© The Author(s) 2018
T. A. Ziegler, *Medieval Healthcare and the Rise of Charitable Institutions*, The New Middle Ages,
https://doi.org/10.1007/978-3-030-02056-9_8

governments allowed for the creation of governmental and public buildings where official healthcare could occur. Leaders, such as the pharaohs of Egypt, constructed temples for worship, and at the temples, religion and healthcare were combined. Temple priests saw to the basic needs of the sick and injured, while gods, such as Imhotep, healed those who remained at the temple through "temple incubation."

The Greek period brought about more sophisticated methods of care. The Greeks widely imitated the Egyptians, adopting the concepts of a healer god—Apollo—and temple incubation. Later, however, Apollo was replaced in the fifth century BCE by the physician, Asclepius. Asclepius was followed by other Greek physicians, namely Hippocrates and Galen. The body of medical knowledge produced by this group was immense, but the care for the sick remained the same: public temples remained the locus of care.

Much of the knowledge of the Greeks was disseminated and adopted by the Romans. The care of the sick, however, regressed in Republican and Imperial Rome. While the Romans were known for their public baths and general concern for their cities—*Amor civicus*—their concern for the sick, especially those of the lower classes, was not a priority. Rather, it was the introduction of Christianity, along with the Christian concepts of loving the poor and caring for the sick—*caritas*—that created some of the greatest contributions to centralized healthcare.

## Christianity and Early Hospitals and Charitable Institutions

The Christian tenant to care for the poor and sick provided the peoples of Late Antiquity with a mission. This mission, coupled with the concept of *Amor civicus*, began a trend to provide where and when one could for those less fortunate. With the decline of the Roman Empire, however, the means to provide fell on those with adequate resources to do so, which meant that, at least in the early Middle Ages, the burden was upon that of the monastery and sometimes secular princes. Perhaps most innovative in this period was the creation of the Basileias in Byzantium, which merged many of the concepts of monastic and public care. Knowledge of this institution was brought into the West after the "Triumph of Orthodoxy," which also saw the end of Byzantine Iconoclasm, and the restoration of icons to the Eastern Church, and the reemergence of discussion, trade, and exchange between the two regions. Later still, new medical advances appeared in Italy, influenced greatly by the Islamic hospitals and medical advances at them.

The monastery was the main care center for those who were sick, injured, or poor in the early Middle Ages; the burden to care for the destitute of society was immense. As the high Middle Ages approached, the encumbrance was lifted, especially in the wake of the Peace of God movements and the lay movement of the *vita apostolica activa*. Wanting to live a life like that of Christ's apostles, lay men and women sought out ways to help the poor and sick. Since they were limited in the ways in which they could help, the peoples of the high Middle Ages returned to an initiative of the Roman period: *Amor civicus*. What better way to show your love for your city and its people than through the donation of moneys and lands for hospitals that would care for the city's downtrodden?

Although much money and land for the creation of hospitals came from the laity, the construction of such institutions was not a strictly lay affair; hospitals in the high Middle Ages were ultimately religious institutions. The production and management of a hospital meant that the church would have to be involved, as many had chapels and were run by those under a Rule. In the age of heterodoxy, the rise of such institutions that straddled the religious–secular divide provoked greater disagreement over who had jurisdiction. The church reasserted its power and sought reform through various local and general councils.

## THE HOSPITAL OF SAINT JOHN IN BRUSSELS: ITS IMPORTANCE

The question of secular–religious divide was never more apparent than it was in Brussels at Saint John hospital. Members of the both secular and lay society originally formed the hospital of Saint John as a confraternity. Its evolution into a hospital was rapid, and its patronage by the local dukes, the town burghers, and even the priesthood called into question who controlled the institution. In 1211, the issue of jurisdiction was made clear when the bishop of Cambrai intervened—the bishop provided the hospital with a set of statutes that solidified the bishop's role, prohibited the role of secular leaders, and reformed the hospital in lieu of recent councils.

The intention of the statutes was to limit the secular control and reform the hospital under the bishop's expertise. It was a return to the role of the bishop as the father of the poor—after all, father knows best!

What occurred, however, after the issuance of Saint John's statutes, proved to be much more remarkable. The battle between religious and secular leaders continued to wage, not only in Brussels but also beyond. As the church fought to assert its power, the hospital, whose bishops were engulfed in the greater Church–Empire war, ended up benefiting significantly. Moreover, the associates of the hospital of Saint John were placed in contact with others who, seeing the benefits associated with the Saint John's statutes, borrowed them and used them in their own dioceses primarily because they addressed the decrees of the reforming councils.

As the Church–Empire debate came to a close, Saint John hospital in Brussels exploded in growth. A campaign for the reconstruction of the hospital emerged in the mid-thirteenth century. Patrons, recognizing the municipal significance of this particular hospital, donated to the hospital and created a permanent patrimony, which in turn secured the hospital's success into the future. By the end of thirteenth century, the hospital of Saint John was *the* municipal hospital of Brussels, built by the people and for the people.

Its success was not singular, but was owed to the many people associated with its creation: Saint John hospital was an amalgam of religious and secular administration, which caused turmoil but also shaped it into the institution that it became by 1300. The hospital, although significant to the people of Brussels, was indeed the city's first municipal hospital, the first general hospital. We tend to associate municipal hospitals with the fourteenth century and the subsequent Protestant Reformation. The separation of church and state and the rise of institutions under state care have, however, limited our awareness of the fact that municipal institutions existed long before the sixteenth century and even before the fourteenth. The municipal hospital was already in existence before the Reformation, and it was certainly functional in the early part of the thirteenth century. Moreover, Saint John hospital is not the only hospital that existed by 1300. We thus need to reevaulate the ways in which we have viewed and classified these institutions.

The hospital of Saint John is not the only piece in the greater puzzle that created the municipal hospital. In the later Middle Ages, subsequent institutions, directed at both charity and healthcare, emerged, especially in Mediterranean Europe.[1] The evolutions that would forge the modern hospital were still to come, but the basis had been put in place. Saint John hospital of Brussels was the one of many municipal hospitals, and although the institution is gone, its influence will forever be memorialized. Its focus on care for all with an eye to reform set the trajectory for other hospitals to be created and laying the basis for today's institution that still continues to question and span the public and private divide.

[1] See, for example, John Henderson, *Piety and Charity in Late Medieval Florence* (Chicago: University of Chicago Press, 1997).

# BIBLIOGRAPHY

*Charters*

*Cartulaire de l'Hôpital Saint-Jean de Bruxelles (Actes des XII<sup>e</sup> et XIII<sup>e</sup> Siècles).*
Edited by Paul Bonenfant. Brussels: Palais des Académies, 1953:
SJ 3, 5, 7, 8, 9, 10, 11, 12, 13, 14, 15, 20, 21, 23, 25, 34, 38, 41, 49, 50, 51, 55, 56, 60, 76, 85, 90, 91, 100, 101, 119, 121, 122, 128, 131, 132, 139-145, 148, 151, 153, 164, 165, 171, 172, 180, 188, 191, 195, 197, 198, 200, 203, 204, 205, 207, 208, 210, 215, 216, 218, 219, 222, 223, 224, 225, 226 227, 229, 241, 249, 250, 251, 253, 254, 256, 259, 260, 261, 262, 263, 264, 266, 267, 269, 270, 271, 275, 276, 277.
Brussels, *Centre Public d'Action Sociale de Bruxelles* (CPAS):
SJ 4.
SJ 4, fol. 1.
SJ 4, fol. 2.
SJ 4, fol. 3.
SJ 4, fol 5.
SJ 4, fol 7.
SJ 4, fol. 11.
SJ 4, fol. 13.
SJ 4, fol. 17.
SJ 4, fol. 18.
SJ 4, fol. 27.
SJ 5.
SJ 31.

© The Editor(s) (if applicable) and The Author(s), under exclusive license to Springer Nature Switzerland AG, part of Springer Nature 2018
T. A. Ziegler, *Medieval Healthcare and the Rise of Charitable Institutions*, The New Middle Ages, https://doi.org/10.1007/978-3-030-02056-9

SJ 35.
SJ 35, fol. 49.
SJ 36.
SJ 36, fol 20.
SJ 36, fol 56.
SJ 37.
SJ 40.
SJ 40, fol 4.
SJ 40, fol. 5.
SJ 45.

## Primary Sources

Abbot Benedict of Peterborough, Gervase of Canterbury, William of Newburgh, and Roger of Hoveden. *Decrees of the Ecumenical Councils*. Edited by Norman P. Tanner. Washington, DC: Georgetown University Press, 1990. http://www.ewtn.com/library/COUNCILS/LATERAN3.HTM.

*Administration Générale des Hospices et Secours de la ville de Bruxelles: Hôpital Saint-Jean*. Brussels: CPAS.

*Analectes pour servir à l'histoire ecclésiastique de la Belgique*, tome 2. Brussels, 1865.

*Analectes pour servir à l'histoire ecclésiastique de la Belgique*, tome 29. Louvain, 1901.

Benedict. *The Holy Rule of St. Benedict*. Translated by Boniface Verheyen, 1949. http://www.kansasmonks.org/RuleOfStBenedict.html#ch4.

*Cartulaire de l'Hôpital Saint-Jean de Bruxelles (Actes des XIIᵉ et XIIIᵉ Siècles)*. Edited by Paul Bonenfant. Brussels: Palais des Académies, 1953.

*Chartes du Chapitre de Sainte-Gudule à Bruxelles 1047–1300*. Edited by P. Lefèvre, Ph. Godding, and F. Godding-Ganshof. Université de Louvain: Leuven and Brussels, 1993.

"Code of Hammurabi." *The Avalon Project*. http://avalon.law.yale.edu/subject_menus/hammenu.asp.

Copho (attributed). "Anatomy of the Pig." *Medieval Italy: Texts in Translation*. Edited by Katherine L. Jansen, Joanna Drell, and Frances Andrews. Philadelphia: University of Pennsylvania Press, 2009.

Diodorus Siculus. *Library of History*, volume 1. *Loeb Classics Online*. http://penelope.uchicago.edu/Thayer/E/Roman/Texts/Diodorus_Siculus/1D*.html.

Documents from the First Council of Nicea [The First Ecumenical Council]. Edited by Henry R. Percival. *The Seven Ecumenical Councils of the Undivided Church*, vol XIV of Nicene and Post Nicene Fathers, 2nd series. Edited by Philip Schaff and Henry Wace. Reprint Edinburgh: T&T Clark; Grand Rapids

MI: Wm.B. Eerdmans, 1988. *Fordham Internet Sourcebook*. http://source-books.fordham.edu/halsall/basis/nicea1.txt.

"Episcopal organization of charitable institutions," 12.10, *Lives of the Holy Fathers of Merida*, 5.3 in *Pagans and Christians in Late Antiquity: A Sourcebook*. Edited by A.D. Lee. New York: Routledge Press, 2000, 225–226.

Galen. *Method of Medicine*. Books 1–4. Edited and translated by Ian Johnston and G.H.R. Horsley. Cambridge: Harvard University Press, 2011.

Glorieux, P. *Répertoire des Maitres en Théologie de Paris au XIII^e siècle*. Paris: Librairie Philosophique J. Vrin, 1934.

Herodotus. *The History of Herodotus*. Book II. Translated by George Rawlinson. http://classics.mit.edu/Herodotus/history.html.

Hippocrates of Cos. *Regimen 1*, 229. *Loeb Classics Online*. https://www.loeb-classics.com/view/hippocrates_cos-regimen_i/1931/pb_LCL150.229.xml.

*The Hippocratic Oath: Text, Translation, and Interpretation*. Translation from the Greek by Ludwig Edelstein. Baltimore: The Johns Hopkins Press, 1943. http://guides.library.jhu.edu/c.php?g=202502&p=1335752.

Hippolytus. *The Apostolic Tradition* of *Hippolytus*. Edited by Gregory Dix. London: SPCK, 1968.

*Inventaires des Archives de la Belique: Chartes et Cartulaires des duchés de Brabant et de Limbourg et des Pays d'Outre-Meuse*. Publiés par ordre du Gouvernement sous la direction de l'Administration des Archives Générales du Royaume. Bruxelles: Hayez, 1910.

Jacobs, Roel. "Plutôt vaste, l'ancien hôpital Saint-Jean." In *La Capitale*, 18 November 2003.

"Lateran IV: Canon Six." *Fordham Internet Sourcebook*. http://sourcebooks.fordham.edu/basis/lateran4.asp.

Masudi. *The Meadows of Gold*. Edited and translated by Paul Lunde and Caroline Stone. New York: Routledge, 2010.

Matthew, Platearus. *Circa instans. Medieval Italy: Texts in Translation*. Edited by Katherine L. Jansen, Joanna Drell, and Frances Andrews. Philadelphia: University of Pennsylvania Press, 2009.

*Pachomian Komonia, Vol.1: The Life of Saint Pachomius and His Disciples*. Translated by Armaund Veilleux. Kalamazoo: Cistercian Publications, 1980.

Peter the Deacon. "Biography of Constantine the African." *Medieval Italy: Texts in Translation*. Edited by Katherine L. Jansen, Joanna Drell, and Frances Andrews. Philadelphia: University of Pennsylvania Press, 2009.

*Quran*. Surah Al-Israa, 17:82. In IqraSense, *Healing and Shifa: From Quran and Sunnah*. Scotts Valley, USA: IqraSense, 2013.

*The Rule of Saint Augustine*. Translated by Robert Russell from Luc Verheijen. *La regle de saint Augustin*. Paris: Etudes Augustiniennes, 1967.

*Statuts d'hotels-Dieu et de léproseries; recueil de textes du XII^e au XIV^e siècle*. Edited par Léon Le Grand. Paris: Alphonse Picard et Fils, 1901.

Tertullian. *Apology* 39.1–6. In A.D. Lee, *Pagans and Christians in Late Antiquity: A Sourcebook*. New York: Routledge Press, 2000.

*The Theodosian Code and Novels and the Sirmondian Constitutions*. Translated by Clyde Pharr. Princeton: Princeton University Press, 1980.

Thomas, Aquinas. *On Love and Charity: Readings from the Commentary on the Sentences of Peter Lombard*. Translated by Peter A. Kwaniewski, Thomas Bolin, and Joseph Bolin. Washington, DC: The Catholic University Press of America, 2008.

Trota (?). "Obstetrical Excerpts from the Salernitan Compendium." In *Medieval Italy: Texts in Translation*. Edited by Katherine L. Jansen, Joanna Drell, and Frances Andrews. Philadelphia: University of Pennsylvania Press, 2009.

Victor of Vita. *History of the Persecution of The Province of Africa*. "The Charity of Deogratias, Bishop of Carthage, to the Captives Brought from Rome by the Vandals," 1.24–6. *Readings in Late Antiquity: A Sourcebook*. Edited by Michal Maas. New York: Routledge, 2000.

### Secondary Sources

*Analectes pour servir à l'histoire ecclésiastique de la Belgique*, tome 2. Brussels, 1865.

*Analectes pour servir à l'histoire ecclésiastique de la Belgique*, tome 29. Louvain, 1901.

d'Anvers, Jean. *Brabantsche Yeesten*. J. F. Williams et J. V. Boendale. *Les Gestes des Ducs de Brabant, par Jean de Klerk, D'Anvers*. Bruxelles: M. Hayéz, 1843.

"Aperçu sur l'Assistance Publique de Bruxelles des origines à la fin de l'Ancien Régime." *le Palotin*, 4 (December 1944): 2–3.

Arnade, Peter J., Martha Howell, and Walter Simons. "Fertile Spaces: the Productivity of Urban Space in Northern Europe." *Journal of Interdisciplinary History* XXXII, no. 4 (Spring 2002): 515–548.

Avalos, Hector. *Illness and Health Care in the Ancient Near East: The Role of the Temple in Greece, Mesopotamia, and Israel*. Atlanta: Scholar Press, 1995.

Barefoot, Peter. "Asklepieia: Ideas for Design Today." In *Health and Antiquity*. Edited by Helen King. New York: Routledge, 2005.

Barguet, P. *La stèle de la famine à Séhel*, volume 34. Paris: Institut français d'archaéologie orientale, 1953.

Bernaerts, Aimé, and Roger Kervyn de Marcke ten Driessche. *Les noms de Rues à Bruxelles: leur histoire—leur signication—leur sort*. Bruxelles: Editions de Vissccher, 1951.

Bettenson, Henry, ed. *Documents of the Christian Church*, 2nd ed. London: Oxford University Press, 1963.

Bischoff, Bernard. *Latin Paleography: Antiquity and the Middle Ages.* Translated by Dáibhí Ó Cróinín and David Ganz. Cambridge: Cambridge University Press, 2007.

Blockmans, W.B. "Urban Space in the Low Countries 13th–16th Centuries." *Spazio urbano e organizzazione economia nell'Europa medieval* [Annali della Facoltà di Scienze Politiche] 29 (Materiali di Storia 14), 1993–1994.

Bonenfant, Paul. "Une capital au berceau: Bruxelles." *Annales: Économies, Sociétés, Civilisations 4ᵉ année* 4, no. 3 (1949): 298–310.

———. *D'Histoire des Hôpitaux.* Brussels: Annales de la Société Belge, 1965.

———. *Le Problème du Paupérisme en Belgique a la fin de l'Ancien Régime.* Bruxelles: Palais des Académies, 1934.

———. "L'origine des villes brabançonnes et la <<route>> de Bruges à Cologne." *Revue belge de philology et d'histoire*, tome 31 fasc. 2–3 (1953).

———. "Les premiers remparts de Bruxelles." *Annales de la Société royale d'archéologie de Bruxelles* XL (1936): 7–47.

———. "Quelques cadres territoriaux de l'histoire de Bruxelles: comté, ammannie, quartier, arrondissement." In *Annales de la Société d'Archéologie de Bruxelles: Mémoires, Rapports et Documents*, tome 39. Bruxelles, 1934.

———. *Saint-Jean de Bruxelles ou Saint-Médard de Soissons? Bulletin de la Commission Royale d'Histoire*, tome XCI. Bruxelles, 1927.

Bonenfant-Feytmans, A.M. "La reception des maladies dans les hôpitaux de Bruxelles avant 1914." Notice historique. In *Archiviste de la Commission d'Assitance publique de Bruxelles.* Bruxelles, 1963.

Boyd, Kenneth M. "Disease, Illness, Sickness, Health, Healing and Wholeness: Exploring Some Elusive Concepts." *Journal of Medical Ethics: Medical Humanities* 26 (2000): 9–17.

Boyle, Leonard E. "Diplomatics." In *Medieval Studies: An Introduction*, 2nd ed. Edited by James M. Powell. Syracuse: Syracuse University Press, 1992.

Breasted, John Henry. *The Edwin Smith Surgical Papyrus.* University of Chicago Press: University of Chicago, 1930.

Broca, Paul. "Sur les Trépanations préhistoriques." *Bull Soc Anthrop* 11: 461–463.

———. "Trépanation chez les Incas." *Bull Acad Méd* (Paris) 32: 866–872.

Brodman, James William. *Charity and Welfare: Hospitals and the Poor in Medieval Catalonia.* The Middle Ages Series. Philadelphia: University of Pennsylvania Press, 1998.

———. *Charity and Religion in Medieval Europe.* Washington, DC: The Catholic University of America Press, 2009.

———. "Religion and Discipline." In *The Medieval Hospital and Medical Practice: AVISTA Studies in the History of Medieval Technology, Science and Art*, volume 3. Edited by Barbara S. Bowers. Burlington: Ashgate, 2007.

Brown, Peter. *The Cult of Saints: Its Rise and Function in Latin Christianity.* Chicago: University of Chicago Press, 1982.

———. *The Making of Late Antiquity.* Cambridge: Harvard University Press, 1978.

———. *Through the Eye of a Needle: Wealth, the Fall of Rome, and the Making of Christianity in the West 350–550 AD.* Princeton: Princeton University Press, 2014.

Brune, Paul. *Histoire de l'ordre Hospitalier du Saint-Esprit.* Paris: C. Martin, 1892.

*Brussels.* Edited by Claire Billen and Jean-Marie Duvosquel. Mercator Fonds: Antwerp, 2000.

*Bruxelles: Croissance d'une capital.* Sous la direction de Jean Stengers, et al. Anvers: Fonds Mercator, 1979.

De Bruyn, H. "Origine de l'Église et de l'hôpital de Saint-Jean, au Marais, a Bruxelles." *Analectes Pour Servir à l'histoire ecclésiastique de la Belgique,* tome 4. Brussels, 1867, 31.

Bryan, P.W. *The Papyrus Ebers.* London: Geoffrey Bles, 1930.

Camille, Michael. "Signs of the City: Place, Power, and Public Fantasy in Medieval Paris." In *Medieval Practices of Space.* Edited by Barbara A. Hanawalt and Michal Kobialka. Minneapolis: University of Minnesota Press, 2000.

Cariboni, Guido. "'No One Can Serve Two Masters': Abbots and Arch-Abbots in the Monastic Networks at the End of the Eleventh Century." *The Journal of Medieval Monastic Studies* 2: 39–74. Edited by Janet Burton and Karen Stöber. Turnhout: Brepols, 2013.

*Cartulaire de l'Hôpital Saint-Jean de Bruxelles (Actes des XIIᵉ et XIIIᵉ Siècles).* Edited by Paul Bonenfant. Brussels: Palais des Académies, 1953.

Charruadas, Paulo. "The Cradle of the City: The Environmental Imprint of Brussels and Its Hinterland in the High Middle Ages." *Regional Environmental Change* 12 (2) (June 2012): 223–238.

———. "Croissance Rurale et Action Seigneuriale aux origines de Bruxelles (Haut Moyen Âge- XIIIᵉ siècle)." *Studies in European Urban History 10 (1100–1800)* "Voisinages, Coexistences, Appropriations: Groupes sociaux et territoires urbains (Moyen Âge-16ᵉ siècle)." Sous la direction de Chloé Deligne et Claire Billen. Turnhout: Brepolis, 2007.

*Chartes du Chapitre de Sainte-Gudule à Bruxelles 1047–1300.* Edited by P. Lefèvre, Ph. Godding, and F. Godding-Ganshof. Université de Louvain: Leuven and Brussels, 1993.

Cherryhomes, Rawlins. "Charity in Brussels: The Hospital Saint John (1186–1300)." Unpublished Masters, University of Texas, 1963.

*Church and City 1000–1500: Essays in Honour of Christopher Brooke.* Edited by David Abulafia, Michael Franklin, and Miri Rubin. Cambridge: Cambridge University Press, 1992.

Clark, Gillian. *Women in Late Antiquity: Pagan and Christian Life-Styles.* Oxford: Clarendon Press, 1993.

Clarke, Helen, and Björn Ambrosiani. *Towns in the Viking Age.* New York: Saint Martin's Press, 1991.

Clay, Rotha Mary. *The Medieval Hospitals of England.* London: Frank Cass & Co., 1966.

LeClercq, Jean, et al. *The Spirituality of the Middle Ages.* New York: Seabury Press, 1982.

*A Companion to Science, Technology, and Medicine in Ancient Greece and Rome,* volume I. Edited by Georgia L. Irby. Oxford: Wiley Blackwell, 2016.

Constable, Giles. *The Reformation of the Twelfth Century.* Cambridge: Cambridge University Press, 1996.

———. *Three Studies in Medieval Religious and Social Thought.* Cambridge: Cambridge University Press, 1998.

Crislip, Andrew T. *From Monastery to Hospital: Christian Monasticism and the Transformation of Health Care in Late Antiquity.* Ann Arbor: The University of Michigan Press, 2005.

Cullum, Patricia. *Cremets and Corrodies: Care of the Poor and Sick at St Leonard's Hospital, York, in the Middle Ages.* York: Borthwick Papers, 1995.

Damen, Mario and Robert Stein. "Collective Memory and Personal *Memoria.* The Carthusian Monastery of Scheut as a Crossroads of Urban and Princely Patronage in Fifteenth Century Brabant." *Mémoires conflictuelles et mythes concurrents dans les pays bourguignons (ca 1380–1580): Rencontres de Luxembourg.* Neuchâtel: Centre Européen d'Études Bourguignonnes (XIVᵉ–XVIᶜ s.), 2012.

Davis, Adam J. "The Social and Religious Meanings of Charity in Medieval Europe." *History Compass* 12, no. 12 (December 2014): 935–950.

Deligne, Chloé. *Bruxelles et sa rivière: Genèse d'un territoire urbain (12ᵉ–18ᵉ siècle).* Turnhout: Brepols, 2003.

———. "Petites villes et grands marchands? Pur une reconsidération de l'histoire des villes Hainuyères (XIIIe siècle -XIVe siècle)." *Studies in European Urban History 10 (1100–1800).* "Voisinages, Coexistences, Appropriations: Groupes sociaux et territoires urbains (Moyen Âge-16ᶜ siècle)." Sous la direction de Chloé Deligne et Claire Billen. Turnhout: Brepolis, 2007.

———. "Powers Over Space, Spaces of Powers. The Constitution of Town Squares in the Cities of the Low Countries (12th–14th Centuries)." *The Power of Space in late Medieval and Early Modern Europe: The Cities of Italy, Northern France and the Low Countries.* Edited by Marc Boone and Martha Howell. Turnhout: Brepols, 2013.

Delisle, Léopold. "Memoires sur les actes d'Innocent III." Dans *Bibliothèque de l'École des chartes,* 4ᶜ série, 4, tome 19, 1858.

Despy, Georges. "Un dossier mystérieux: les origins de Bruxelles." *Bulletin de la Classe des Lettres et des Science Morales et Politiques*, 6ᵉ série, tome VIII. Bruxelles: Académie Royale de Belgique, 1997.

———. "La genese d'une ville." In Jean Stengers et al., *Bruxelles: Croissance d'une capital.* Anvers: Fonds Mercator, 1979.

Devroey, Jean-Pierre. "Twixt Meuse and Scheldt: Town and Country in the Medieval Economy of the Southern Netherlands from the Sixth to the Twelfth Century." *The Fascinating Faces of Flanders: Through Art and Society.* Translated from French by Van Lokeren. Anvers: City of Antwerp, 1998.

Dickstein-Bernard, Claire. "Activité économique et développement urbain à Bruxelles (XIIIᵉ–XVᵉ siècles)." *Cahiers Bruxellois* 24 (1979): 52–62.

Duby, Georges. *The Early Growth of the European Economy: Warriors and Peasants from the Seventh to the Twelfth Century.* Ithaca: Cornell University Press, 1978.

———. "Taking, Giving and Consecrating." In *The Early Growth of the European Economy.* Translated by Howard B. Clarke. Ithaca, NY: Cornell University Press, 1974.

Dunn, Marilyn. *The Emergence of Monasticism: From the Desert Fathers to the Early Middle Ages.* Oxford: Blackwell, 2003.

Duparc, Pierre. "Confraternities of the Holy Spirit and Village Communities in the Middle Ages." In *Lordship and Community in Medieval Europe: Selected Readings.* Edited and translated by Fredric L. Cheyette. Huntington: Robert E. Krieger Publishing, 1975.

Durham, Brian. "The Infirmary and Hall of the Medieval Hospital of St John the Baptist." *Oxoniensia* 56 (1992): 17–75.

Evrard, Paul. "Formation, organization generale et etat du domaine rural de l'hôpital Saint Jean au Moyen-Age." Unpublished Master's Thesis, Universite Libre de Bruxelles, 1965.

Farmer, Sharon. "Down and Out and Female in Thirteenth-Century Paris." *The American Historical Review* 103, no. 2 (April 1998): 345–372.

———. "From Personal Charity to Centralised Poor Relief: The Evolution of Responses to the Poor in Paris, c. 1250–1600." In *Experiences of Charity.* Edited by Anne M. Scott. Burlington: Ashgate, 2015.

———. *Surviving Poverty in Medieval Paris: Gender, Ideology, and the Daily Lives of the Poor.* Ithaca: Cornell University Press, 2002, 2005.

Favresse, Félicien. *Etudes sur les métiers bruxellois au moyen âge.* Bruxelles: Université libre de Bruxelles Institut de Sociologie, 1961.

Ferngren, Gary. "The Sick Poor and the Origins of Medical Charity." Available Online at http://chreader.org/sick-poor-origins-medical-charity/.

Ferguson, Everett. *Backgrounds of Early Christianity.* Grand Rapids: William B. Eerdmans, 1993.

BIBLIOGRAPHY 143

Foucault, Michel. *The Birth of the Clinic: An Archaeology of Mediecal Perception.* Translated by A.M. Sheridan Smith. New York: Vintage Books, 1994.

———. "La politique de la santé au XVIIIe siècle." *Les Machines à guérir, Aux origines de l'hôpital moderne*; dossiers et documents. Paris: Institut de l'environnement, 1976.

Gautier, Paul. "Le typikon du Christ Sauveur Pantocrator." *REB* 32 (1974): 1–145.

Geary, Patrick J. *Living with the Dead in the Middle Ages.* Ithaca: Cornell University Press, 1994.

*Gestes des Èvêques de Cambrai de 1092–1138.* Edited by Charles de Smedt et S.J. Bollandiste. Paris: Librairie Renouard, 1880.

Gilliat-Smith, Ernest. *Story of Brussels.* London: J.M. Dent, 1906.

Glorieux, P. *Répertoire des Maitres en Théologie de Paris au XIIIᵉ siècle.* Librairie Philosophique J. Vrin: Paris, 1934.

Goyau, Georges. "Councils of Orléans." *The Catholic Encyclopedia*, volume 11. New York: Robert Appleton Company, 1911. http://www.newadvent.org/cathen/11318a.htm.

Le Grand, Léon. *Statuts d'hotels-Dieu et de léproseries; recueil de textes du XIIᵉ au XIVᵉ siècle.* Paris: Alphonse Picard et Fils, 1901.

Green, Monica H. "Gendering the History of Women's Healthcare." *Gender & History* 20, no. 3 (2008): 487–518.

———. "'History of Medicine' or 'History of Health'." *Past and Future*, no. 9 (Spring/Summer 2011): 7.

———. *Making Women's Medicine Masculine: The Rise of Male Authority in Premodern Gynaecology.* Oxford: Oxford University Press, 2008.

Hajar, R. "Learning Ancient Greek Medicine from Homer." *Heart Views* 3 (2002): 8.

Haskins, Charles Homer. *The Renaissance of the Twelfth Century.* Cambridge: Harvard University Press, 1927.

Henderson, John. *Piety and Charity in Late Medieval Florence.* Chicago: University of Chicago Press, 1997.

Henne, Alexandre et Alphonse Wauters. *Histoire de la Ville de Bruxelles.* Bruxelles: Perichon, 1845, 1968.

Hinnebush, John Frederick. *The Historia Occidentalis of Jacques de Vitry: A Critical Edition.* Fribourg: The University Press, 1972.

*The Hospital in History.* Edited by Lindsay Granshaw and Roy Porter. New York: Routledge,1989.

Howell, Martha C. "The Spaces of Late Medieval Urbanity." In *Shaping Urban Identity in Late Medieval Europe.* Edited by Marc Boone and Peter Stabel. Leuven-Apeldoorn: Garant, 2000.

Imbert, Jean. *Histoire des hôpitaux francais.* Paris: J. Vrin, 1947.

IqraSense. *Healing and Shifa: From Quran and Sunnah*. Scotts Valley, USA: IqraSense, 2013.

Jansen, Katherine Ludwig. *The Making of the Magdalen: Preaching and Popular Devotion in the Later Middle Ages*. Princeton: Princeton University Press, 2000.

Jonson, Albert R. *A Short History of Medical Ethics*. Oxford: Oxford University Press, 2000.

Kealey, Edward. "Hospitals and Poor Relief, Western Europe." *Dictionary of the Middle Ages*. Edited by Joseph Strayer. New York: Charles Scribner's Sons, 1989.

———. *Medieval Medicus: A Social History of Anglo-Norman Medicine*. Baltimore: The John Hopkins University Press, 1981.

Kleinman, Arthur. *Patients and Healers in the Context of Culture. An Exploration of the Borderland Between Anthropology, Medicine, and Psychiatry*. Berkeley: University of California Press, 1980.

Kusman, David. "*Domos suas ou in domo Lombardorum?* Les strategies d'implantation urbaine des communautes marchandes piemontaises: le cas du Duche de Brabant (XIIIᵉ siècle–XVᵉ siècle)." *Studies in European Urban History 10 (1100–1800)*. "Voisinages, Coexistences, Appropriations: Groupes sociaux et territoires urbains (Moyen Âge-16ᵉ siècle)." Sous la direction de Chloé Deligne et Claire Billen. Turnhout: Brepolis, 2007.

Kwaniewski, Peter. In Thomas Aquinas, *On Love and Charity: Readings from the Commentary on the Sentences of Peter Lombard*. Translated by Peter A. Kwaniewski, Thomas Bolin, and Joseph Bolin. Washington, DC: The Catholic University Press of America, 2008.

Labat, René. *Traité akkadien de diagnostics et prognostics médicaux*. Paris: Academie Internationale d'Historie des Sciences, 1951.

Lallemand, Léon. *La lèper et lèproseries du Xᵉ au XVIᵉ siècles* in *Compte rendu des séances de l'Academie des sciences morales et politiques*—N.S. LxIII, CLXIIIᵉ de la Collection. Paris, 1905.

Lee, A.D. *Pagans and Christians in Late Antiquity: A Sourcebook*. New York: Routledge Press, 2000.

LeFebvre, Henri. *The Production of Space*. Translated by Donald Nicholson-Smith. Malden: Blackwell, 1991.

Lilley, K.D. *Urban Life in the Middle Ages: 1000–1450*. New York: Palgrave, 2002.

Lillich, Meredith Parsons. "The Choir Clerestory Windows of La Trinité at Vendôme: Dating and Patronage." *The Journal of the Society of Architectural Historians* 34, no. 3 (October 1975): 238–250.

Lindberg, Carter. *Beyond Charity: Reformation Initiatives for the Poor*. Minneapolis: Augsburg Fortress, 1993.

———. *Love: A Brief History Through Western Christianity.* Oxford: Blackwell, 2008.

Little, Lester K. *Religious Poverty and the Profit Economy in Medieval Europe.* Ithaca: Cornell University Press, 1978.

Lynch, Kevin. *The Image of the City.* Cambridge: The M.I.T. Press, 1960.

des Marez, G. "Le développement territorial de Bruxelles ua Moyen age." In *Congrés International de Géographie Historique*, tome III, Bruxelles: Falk fils, 1935.

Martens, Mina. *Histoire de Bruxelles.* Brussels: Privat, 1976.

_____. *L'Administration du Domaine Ducal en Brabant au Moyen-Âge (1250–1406).* Brussels: Académie Royale de Belgique, 1952.

———. "Du site rural au site semi-urbain." In *Histoire de Bruxelles.* Toulouse: Privat, 1976.

Marx, Walter John. *The Development of Charity in Medieval Louvain.* New York: Yonkers, 1936.

Mauss, Marcel. *The Gift: Forms and Functions of Exchange in Archaic Societies.* Translated by Ian Cunnison. New York: Norton, 1967.

*The Medieval Hospital and Medical Practice: AVISTA Studies in the History of Medieval Technology, Science and Art*, volume 3. Edited by Barbara S. Bowers. Burlington: Ashgate, 2007.

*Medieval Italy: Texts in Translation.* Edited by Katherine L. Jansen, Joanna Drell, and Frances Andrews. Philadelphia: University of Pennsylvania Press, 2009.

*Medieval Practices of Space.* Edited by Barbara A. Hanawalt and Michal Kobialka. Minneapolis: University of Minnesota Press, 2000.

"Medievalism and the Medical Humanities." Edited by Jamie McKinstry and Corinne Saunders. *Postmedieval: A Journal of Medieval Cultural Studies* 8 (2017): 139–146.

Melvill, Gert. *The World of Medieval Monasticism: Its History and Forms of Life.* Collegeville: Liturgical Press, 2016.

Milis, Ludo J.R. *Religion, Culture, and Mentalities in the Medieval Low Countries: Selected Essays.* Edited by Jeroen Deploige, Martine De Reu, Walter Simons, and Steven Vanderputten. Belgium: Brepols, 2005.

Miller, Timothy. *The Birth of the Hospital in the Byzantine Empire.* Baltimore: Johns Hopkins University Press, 1985.

Mollat, Michel. *The Poor in the Middle Ages: An Essay in Social History.* Translated by Authur Goldhammer. New Haven: Yale University Press, 1986.

Montford, Angela. *Health, Sickness, Medicine and the Friars in the Thirteenth and Fourteenth Centuries.* Vermont: Ashgate, 2004.

Moore, Norman. *The History of St. Bartholomew's Hospital*, volumes I and II. London: C. Arthur Pearson, 1918.

Moore, R.I. *The Formation of a Persecuting Society.* Oxford, MA: Blackwell, 1990.

de Moreau, S.J.É. *Histoire de l'église en Belgique*, 2ᶜ edition, tomes I–IV. Brussels: L'Édition Universelle, 1945.

Mumford, Lewis. *The City in History. Its Origins, Its Transformations, and Its Prospects.* London: Mariner Books, 1991 (reprint).

*Mummies, Disease, and Ancient Cultures.* Edited by Aiden and Eve Cockburn. Cambridge University Press: Cambridge, 1980.

*National Library of Medicine.* "Islamic Culture and the Medical Arts: Hospitals." https://www.nlm.nih.gov/exhibition/islamic_medical/islamic_12.html.

Newman, Martha G. *The Boundaries of Charity: Cistercian Culture and Ecclesiastical Reform, 1098–1180.* Stanford: Stanford University Press, 1996.

Nicolas, David. *The Growth of the Medieval City: From Late Antiquity to the Early Fourteenth Century.* New York: Routledge, 1997, 2014.

———. *Medieval Flanders.* New York: Longman, 1992.

———. *Urban Europe: 1100–1700.* New York: Palgrave Macmillan, 2003.

Nunn, J.F. *Ancient Egyptian Medicine.* Norman: University of Oklahoma Press, 1996.

Ockeley, Jaak. *De gasthuiszusters en hun ziekenzorg in het aartsbisdom Mechelen in de 17de en de 18de eeuw: deel 1.* Brussel: Algemeen Rijksarchief, 1992.

———. "Ziekenzorg te Brussel van de 12de tot de 19de eeuw, inzonderheid in het Sint- Jansgasthuisop-de-Poel." In *Momenten uit de geschiedenis van Brussel.* Brussels: Centrum Brabantse Geschiedenis, 2000.

Oldfather, Charles Henry. "General Introduction." In Diodorus Siculus, *Library of History*, volume 1. Loeb Classics Online. http://penelope.uchicago.edu/Thayer/E/Roman/Texts/Diodorus_Siculus/1D*.html.

d'Osta, Jean. *Dictionnaire historique et anecdotique des Rues de Bruxelles.* Bruxelles: Paul Legrain, 1986.

———. *Les rues disparues de Bruxelles.* Belgique: Rossel, 1979.

Paxton, Frederick S. *Christianizing Death: The Creation of a Ritual Process in Early Medieval Europe.* Ithaca: Cornell University Press, 1996.

*Poverty and Prosperity in the Middle Ages and Renaissance.* Edited by Cynthia Kosso and Anne Scott. Turnout: Brepols, 2013.

Pirenne, Henri. *Histoire de la Belgique.* Bruxelles: Lamertin, 1902.

———. *Medieval Cities: Their Origins and the Revival of Trade.* Translated by Frank D. Halsey. Princeton: Princeton University Press, 1925, 1969, 1975.

Prioreschi, Plinio. *A History of Medicine: Volume III, Roman Medicine.* Omaha: Horatius Press, 1998.

———. "Possible Reasons for Neolithic Skull Trephining." *Prespectives in Biology and Medicine* 34, no. 2 (Winter 1991): 296–303.

Rawcliffe, Carole. *Medicine and Society in Later Medieval England.* Phoenix Mill: Alan Sutton Publishing, 1995.

Reicke, Siegfried. *Das deutsche Spital und sein Recht im Mittelalter.* Stuttgart: Enke, 1932.

*Religion and Medicine in the Middle Ages.* Edited by Peter Biller and Joseph Ziegler. York: York Medieval Press, 2001.

Reymond, M. "Les Confreries du Saint Esprit au pays de Vaud." *Zeitschrift fur Schweizerische Kirchengeschichte* XX (1926): 282–301.

Rosenwein, Barbara H. *Emotional Communities in the Early Middle Ages.* Ithaca: Cornell University Press, 2006.

Rubin, Miri. *Charity and Community in Medieval Cambridge.* Cambridge: Cambridge University Press, 1987.

*The Rule of Saint Augustine.* Translated by Robert Russell from Luc Verheijen, *La regle de saint Augustin.* Paris: Etudes Augustiniennes, 1967.

Runciman, Steven. *A History of the Crusades,* volume II. Cambridge University Press, 1952.

Said, Hakim Mohammed. *Traditional Greco-Arabic and Modern Western Medicine: Conflict or Symbiosis?* Karachi: Hamdard Academy, 1975.

Schaefer, F.F. *Das hospital zum hl. Geist auf dem Domhofe zu Köln.* Köln: Kreuznach, 1910.

*Shaping Urban Identify in Late Medieval Europe.* Edited by Marc Boone and Peter Stabel. Leuven-Apeldoorn: Garant, 2000.

*A Short History of Medicine.* Edited by Erwin H. Ackerknecht and Lisa Haushofer. Baltimore: John Hopkins University Press, 2016.

Simons, Walter. *Cities of Ladies.* Pennsylvania: University of Pennsylvania Press, 2003.

Siraisi, Nancy. *Medieval and Early Renaissance Medicine: An Introduction to Knowledge and Practice.* Chicago: University of Chicago Press, 1990.

De Smedt, R.P. CH. "L'ordre hospitalier du Saint-Esprit." *Revue des questiones historiques* 54 (1 July 1893): 216–225.

Smets, G. *Henri I Duc de Brabant 1190–1235.* Bruxelles: Lamertine, 1908.

Smith, C.T. *An Historical Geography of Western Europe Before 1800,* rev. ed. New York: Longman, 1967, 1978.

Smith, Ernest. *The Story of Brussels.* Didactic Press, Kindle Edition, 2014.

Snook, Donald Jr. *Hospitals: What They Are and How They Work.* Frederick, MD: Aspen Publishers, 1992.

de Spiegeler, Pierre. *Les Hôpitaux et l'Assistance à Liège ($X^e$–$X^{ve}$ Siècles): Aspects Institutionnels et Sociaux.* Paris: Sociéte d'Edition "Les Belles Lettres," 1987.

Stabel, Peter. "The Market Place and Civic Identity in Late Medieval Flanders." In *Shaping Urban Identity in Late Medieval Europe.* Edited by Marc Boone and Peter Stabel. Leuven: Apeldoorn, 2000.

State, Paul F. *Historical Dictionary of Brussels.* New York: Rowman and Littlefield, 2015.

Steffens, Sven. "Volksnamen in de stad gisteren en vandaag: het geval Sint-Jans- Molenbeek/Urban Popular Place Names Past and Present: The Case of Molenbeek-Saint- Jean/Sint-Jans-Molenbeek." *Brussels Studies* no. 9 (2007).

*Studies in European Urban History 10 (1100–1800)*. "Voisinages, Coexistences, Appropriations: Groupes sociaux et territories urbains (Moyen Âge-16e siècle)." Sous la direction de Chloé Deligne et Claire Billen. Turnhout: Brepolis, 2007.

Thompson, John D., and Grace Goldin. *The Hospital: A Social and Architectural History*. New Haven: Yale University Press, 1975.

*Le Troisième Concile de Latran (1179): San place dans l'histoire*. Communications présentées à la Table Ronde du C.N.R.S. Paris: Études Augustiniennes, 1982.

Vannieuwenhuyze, Bram. *The Study and Classification of Medieval Urban Toponymy: The Case of Late Medieval Brussels (13th–16th Centuries)*. Leuven: Onoma, 2007.

Vannieuwenhuyze, Bram, Paulo Charruadas, Yannick Devos, and Luc Vrydaghs. "The Medieval Territory of Brussels: A Dynamic Landscape of Urbanization." In *Landscape Archeology Between Art and Science*. Edited by S.J. Kluiving and E.B. Guttermann-Bond (2012): 223–238.

Van Schaïk, R. "On the Social Position of Jews and Lombards in the Towns of the Low Countries and Neighboring German Territories During the Late Middle Ages." In *Coeur et marge dans la société urbaine au bas Moyen Âge*, Acts du colloque tenu à Gand (22–23 août 1996). Edited by Carlier, Greve, Prevenier, et Stabel. Louvian-Apeldoorn, 1997.

Vauchez, André. *The Laity in the Middle Ages: Religious Beliefs and Devotional Practices*. Notre Dame: University of Notre Dame Press, c. 1993.

———. *The Spirituality of the Medieval West from the Eighth to the Twelfth Century*. Translated by Colette Friedlander. Kalamazoo: Cistercian Publications, 1993.

Venarde, Bruce L. *Women's Monasticism and Medieval Society: Nunneries in France and England, 890–1215*. Ithaca: Cornell University Press, 1997.

Vercauteren, Fernand. *Actes des Comtes de Flandre 1071–1128*. Bruxelles: Palais des Academies, 1938.

Verhulst, Adriaan. *The Rise of Cities in North-West Europe*. Cambridge: Cambridge University Press, 1999.

Volk, Robert. *Gesundheitswesen und Woltätigkeit im Spiegel der byzantinischedn Klostertypika*. Miscellanea Byzantina Monacensia, 28. Munich: Institut für Byzantinisik, neugriechische Philologie, und byzantinische Kunstgeschichte der Universität Müchen, 1983.

de Vries, André. *Brussels: A Cultural and Literary History*. Oxford: Signal Books, 2003.

Wauters, Alphonse. *Bruxelles et ses environs*. Brussels, 1855.

———. "L'Architecture Romane dans ses diverses transformations." In *Annales de la Société d'Archéologie de Bruxelles: Mémoires, Rapports et Documents*, tome 3. Bruxelles, 1889.

————. *Histoire des Environs de Bruxelles: Description historique des localités qui formaient autrefois l'Ammannie de cette ville*, tomes 1–3. Bruxelles: Impression Anastaltique, 1855, 1968.

————. "Les plus anciens échevins de la Ville de Bruxelles. Essai d'une liste complète de ses magistrats pour les temps antérieurs à l'année 1339. Bruxelles, *Annales de la Société d'Archéologie de Bruxelles*, 1895.

Webb, John L. "The Oldest Medical Document." *Bulletin of the Medical Library Association* 45, no. 1 (January 1957): 1–4.

Weber, Max. *The City*. New York: Free Press, 1958.

White, Stephen D. *Custom, Kinship, and Gifts to Saints: The Laudatio Parentum in Western France, 1050–1150*. Chapel Hill: The University of North Carolina Press, 1988.

Wightman, Edith Mary. *Gallia Belgica*. Berkeley: University of California Press, 1985.

Winch, Michael. *Introducing Belgium*. London: Methuen & Co., 1964.

*With Us Always: A History of Private Charity and Public Welfare*. Edited by Donald T. Critchlow and Charles H. Parker. Lanham: Rowman and Littlefield, 1998.

*Women in Medieval Society*. Edited by Susan Mosher Stuard. Philadelphia: University of Pennsylvania Press, 1976, 1977.

Wölfel, D.J. "Die Trepanation." *Anthropos, Bd* 20 (1925): 1–50.

Ziegler, Tiffany A. "Considering Networks of Charity: Family Traditions, Female Donation Practices, and the Hospital of Saint John's in Brussels." *The Journal of Medieval Prosopography* 29 (2015): 51–74.

————. "'I Was Sick and You Visited Me:' The Hospital of Saint John in Brussels and Its Patrons." Unpublished Ph.D. Dissertation, University of Missouri-Columbia, 2010.

# INDEX

© The Editor(s) (if applicable) and The Author(s), under exclusive license   151
to Springer Nature Switzerland AG, part of Springer Nature 2018
T. A. Ziegler, *Medieval Healthcare and the Rise of Charitable Institutions*,
The New Middle Ages, https://doi.org/10.1007/978-3-030-02056-9

Printed in the USA
CPSIA information can be obtained
at www.ICGtesting.com
CBHW071011280624
10806CB00005B/238